# PHYSICIAN'S GUIDE
## TO SURVIVING
# CGCAHPS
# & HCAHPS

---

## TRINA E. DORRAH, MD, MPH

ISBN: 1495292614
ISBN 13: 9781495292613
Library of Congress Control Number: 2014901335
CreateSpace Independent Publishing Platform
North Charleston, South Carolina

# Dedication

*To my amazing parents: Mom and Dad, I love you so much!
Thank you for your unyielding support of me throughout my life.
You are the best parents a girl could ever have!*

*To my beautiful sister, Millicent: I love you! You are one of the wisest people I know,
and I feel blessed to have you as a sister. You always know the right things to say,
and I appreciate your wisdom and guidance.*

*To Corey, Caleb, Caden, Christian, and Carson: I love you.
Thanks for keeping things fun.*

*To Rodney Puplampu, my husband and the love of my life: Thank you for everything.
Your love and encouragement are greatly appreciated.*

*To my Baylor Scott and White family, past and present: Thanks for making this one
of the best jobs ever. I especially want to thank Dr. Dudley Baker, Dr. Clyde "Bud"
Chumbley, Dr. Rob Watson, Dr. Robyn Buckley, Dr. Tiffany Berry, Mr. Ernie Bovio,
Mrs. Colleen Sundquist, and Mrs. Joy Zimmerman Bodi. All of you have gone out of
your way to support me in some way along this journey, and I thank you. I also want to
thank my colleagues on the patient satisfaction committee, who have encouraged me in
this pursuit: Dr. Andrejs Avots-Avotins, Dr. Michael Reis, Dr. Stephen Sibbitt,
Mrs. Julie Konichek, and Mrs. Robin Marriott.*

*To my patients: You continue to inspire me to be a better physician every day.
This book is dedicated to you.*

# CONTENTS

# Foreword

I may be in the minority, but I love patient satisfaction! In fact, I feel working to improve the patient experience is one of the most rewarding parts of my job.

I started this journey through my work as medical director of quality at my local hospital. My hospital's leadership decided to make patient satisfaction a priority, and they asked me to work with our providers to improve their scores. One thing I quickly realized was that the providers who scored poorly on our patient satisfaction surveys were not always bad providers. In fact, I would have no problem having most of them as my own personal physician. The key differentiator between them and our high performers was that they had trouble connecting with their patients. I started to notice the little things a provider does that make a huge difference for patients. *How* a provider says something is more important than *what* he or she says. Small gestures that show patients a provider cares are viewed equally with clinical skills.

As I continued to shadow more providers, I developed a desire to share what I was learning. I often interact with providers who are frustrated and demoralized by their patient satisfaction results. Some providers have even expressed a desire to leave medicine altogether. That is exactly why I wrote this book. I believe that, like me, most providers go into medicine with a desire to help others. Unfortunately, the culture of patient satisfaction surveys has an unintended consequence of making providers feel that patients are their adversaries. It is my hope that this book will change that.

Throughout this book, I have highlighted simple yet effective strategies that providers can use to improve patient satisfaction. I believe having satisfied patients and families makes medicine more enjoyable. I hope that as you read this book and implement its techniques, you rediscover any passion for health care that has been lost and reconnect with the joy that practicing medicine brings.

Sincerely,
Dr. Trina E. Dorrah

# Prologue

It's Monday morning, and you are headed to the office. As you drive, you mentally run through your day. You have twenty-five patients scheduled, a few of whom are new visits. You have a meeting over lunch, and you desperately need to finish in time to make it to your child's soccer game. Somehow, over the next few hours, you have to see your patients, review labs, answer messages, make follow-up phone calls, and complete your documentation. Sound familiar? What if I told you that in the midst of this chaos, you must also focus on patient satisfaction? I can only imagine the look you would give me. The reality is that this is the world in which health-care providers now live.

Fast-forward a few hours. Your morning has passed effortlessly. It is now time for your one-o'clock appointment. She is a new patient with diabetes, high blood pressure, and high cholesterol. You think to yourself, *How difficult can this be?* Thirty minutes later, you exit the room, feeling upset and frustrated. Despite your best effort, you simply could not establish a good rapport with her. By the end of the visit, you feel certain she will request another provider. Your concerns are later validated when your office manager stops by to tell you she requested a different doctor. If this patient had simply been upset by your failure to meet an unreasonable demand (such as prescribe unnecessary narcotics), you would not be concerned. However, that was not the case. Several patients have requested another provider because they did not feel you were the right fit for them. A trend has started, and you recognize it as such. Unfortunately, you are not sure what to do about it.

You have been with the clinic for two years, and this has only recently become a problem. A few months ago, your clinic decided to focus more attention on patient satisfaction by introducing a patient satisfaction survey. To help with accountability, your medical director now posts all providers' satisfaction data in the break room. You consistently have lower scores than your colleagues. This upsets you because you feel your hard work and dedication to your patients goes unrecognized. You detest the patient satisfaction surveys, but your clinic has made it clear that due to health-care trends, they are here to stay. There is no getting around the survey, so you decide you must learn to deal with it.

Determined to improve, you open your copy of this book and begin to read…

# Introduction

Patient satisfaction. These words make most providers cringe. We know it is impossible to please everyone, so why even try? No matter what we do, there will always be dissatisfied patients. As a provider—whether you are a doctor, a physician assistant, a nurse practitioner, or in a similar profession—you are an expert in your field. You spent years learning your profession. When you interact with patients, you draw on your knowledge and training to make health-care decisions. You know that what is best clinically does not always make your patients happy. For example, no one loves being told that he or she needs to cut out the fried food and start exercising. Yet this is exactly what so many of our patients need. They may not be excited to hear it, but we know it is in their best interest to follow our advice.

Throughout the history of medicine, providers have mainly been asked to focus on patient care. It is your job to diagnose and treat, and everything else is secondary. Even though you want your patients to like you, you may not spend a lot of time thinking about patient satisfaction. In recent years, health care has started to undergo a transformation. Patients and payers are no longer satisfied with providers who are simply good clinicians. The concept of having a good bedside manner has come to the forefront. As patient satisfaction infiltrates health care, providers must respond by extending their focus beyond clinical care. Providers are now being asked to think of their patients as customers and consider their satisfaction with the care experience. This is a paradigm shift for most providers. The momentum to incorporate patient satisfaction is growing. As a provider, what are you to do? Give up? Throw in the towel? Find a new profession? Even though you may occasionally want to answer *yes*, most of us still have a passion for medicine. We entered this profession with a desire to heal. The things we dislike about our jobs often have little to do with our patients and more to do with the frustrations of health care. We want to have amicable relationships with our patients, because that makes our work more enjoyable.

Before we go further, let me give you a little background about myself. I am an internal medicine physician who practices as a hospitalist. I have a passion for patient satisfaction. I love learning about it, and I love teaching it to others. When I was in medical school, we did not talk about the patient experience. We did not discuss patient satisfaction surveys or learn any tools or tips for improving patient satisfaction. My residency was no different. Although we frequently spoke about compassion and empathy, we never discussed the patient experience and our role in improving it. Following residency, I completed a fellowship in quality improvement. This fellowship increased my interest in improving broken processes and systems. Once I began working, I transitioned into my current role in quality, and as part of this role, I began helping providers improve their patient satisfaction.

I quickly realized that the process for teaching providers about patient satisfaction is broken. Like me, most never received formal training on improving the patient experience. As I continued to work with providers, I noticed three consistent traits. First, I noticed that virtually every provider I worked with was an excellent clinician. I would have no problem sending my family to see most of these providers, despite their low patient satisfaction scores. This taught me **Lesson #1**: being a nice person and a good clinician does not always translate to high patient satisfaction scores. Next,

I realized providers were almost unanimous in their desire to improve. We take our profession seriously, so learning that patients are dissatisfied with our care feels like a personal insult. We want to improve because we want our patients to like us. Having a good relationship with our patients is one of the most rewarding aspects of practicing medicine. This taught me **Lesson #2**: despite frustration with the survey, providers value their patients' opinions and are willing to work to improve their satisfaction. Finally, low patient satisfaction scores frustrated almost every provider I worked with. Low scores feel like a personal attack, and the frustration increases when providers are ill equipped to change. This taught me **Lesson #3**: it is unfair to expect a provider to change without offering them the education and tools. All of these lessons encouraged me to write this book. I knew if my providers felt disheartened, many other providers throughout the country felt the same way. My goal for writing this book is to share with you some of the things I have learned. You can think of me as your personal patient satisfaction improvement coach.

You may wonder why so much attention is being focused on patient satisfaction. You may even question why someone would take the time to write an entire book on the subject. The answer is simple: I love the concepts related to patient satisfaction! In addition, I am a physician who is passionate about helping other providers. Health care is changing, and I do not want you to be surprised or ambushed when the changes take effect. We live in a society that focuses on customer service and loyalty.[1] Health care is simply following that trend. Through the growth of social media, it is incredibly easy for your patients to post reviews about you and your practice online. Another stimulus for change is the fact that patient satisfaction is increasingly linked to reimbursement. This is already happening in the hospital setting through value-based purchasing. Using the Consumer Assessment of Healthcare Providers and Systems (CAHPS®) Hospital Survey as the framework (hereinafter referred to as H-CAHPS), a portion of a hospital's reimbursement is tied to how well it performs on the H-CAHPS patient satisfaction survey. This practice has reached the outpatient setting via the Consumer Assessment of Healthcare Providers and Systems (CAHPS®) Clinician & Group Survey (hereinafter referred to as CG-CAHPS).[2]

Tying outpatient reimbursement to patient satisfaction is the next step for a health-care industry that is increasingly focused on customer service. This will happen through the physician value-based payment modifier. The physician value-based payment modifier is an initiative by which your payment as a physician is altered based on how well you perform on certain quality and patient satisfaction measures. The ultimate goal of the physician value-based payment modifier program is for doctors with lower quality and patient satisfaction scores to be paid less than those doctors with higher scores. It is pay-for-performance, and if your performance is subpar, your pay will decrease. CG-CAHPS is important because this is the survey the Centers for Medicare & Medicaid Services (CMS) has chosen to measure patient satisfaction. All providers who participate in fee-for-service Medicare will be required to use the CG-CAHPS survey. Thus, you must understand CG-CAHPS and how to improve your patient satisfaction scores if you do not want to risk declining reimbursement through the value-based payment modifier program.[3]

An important thing to note is that the physician value-based payment modifier is not optional. According to the Affordable Care Act, CMS must apply a value-based payment modifier to reimbursement by 2015. The program initially begins with larger groups of physicians (>100), but as early as 2017, the value-based payment modifier will apply to all physicians who participate in fee-for-service Medicare.[3]

Given the demands of health care, providers feel overwhelmed at the thought of additional work. Providers want to improve, but they do not have time to research the techniques or read lengthy instructional manuals. That is exactly why I wrote this book. This book will help you learn and incorporate key patient satisfaction concepts. I know your time is valuable, so I purposely designed this book to be short. You should be able to complete it over one or two lunch breaks, and the best part is that it is filled with useful tips that are easy to implement. In fact, you can begin applying the majority of these tools as soon as you finish this book. As your personal patient satisfaction improvement coach, there are two things I require from you before we begin. First, you must commit to reading this book. If you do not read the book, how can you possibly hope to apply the concepts? Placing it on your bookshelf or using it as a coaster will not work. Simply reading the book without taking action will not get you the results you want either. Thus, the second thing I require from you is that you implement what you learn. Regardless of your personal feelings about the techniques, **use at least one tool with every patient, every time.** Can you commit to doing these two things? If so, you are ready to begin!

Now for an important disclaimer: the concepts you will learn throughout this book are not novel. In fact, you have probably heard them before. It is rare, however, to find all of the tools in one specific place. This book brings together many of the concepts you have heard before in an easily accessible format. When I teach providers this information, they often say, "Trina, this is common sense." They are absolutely correct. However, common sense is not always as common as we think. Even though we intuitively know what to do, we often do not do it. That is why this book is helpful. All of the tips and tools you need to succeed are here.

This book is designed to help you improve your patient satisfaction. More specifically, it is designed to teach you how to succeed with the CG-CAHPS and H-CAHPS patient satisfaction surveys. Even though this book is written around the framework of these two surveys, the improvement tips are universal. When you think about it, your patients are already reviewing you every day. Through word of mouth, online rating websites, blogs, and social media, your patients are already expressing their opinions about you and your practice. You cannot control this, but what you can do is learn tips to improve the likelihood that those patients leave your health-care facility satisfied. This book will help you get closer to that goal.

CHAPTER 1
# CG-CAHPS Explained

CG-CAHPS is a patient experience survey created by the Agency for Healthcare Research and Quality (AHRQ). It is designed to measure patient perceptions of care in the office setting. Although it was developed by AHRQ, Medicare has adopted and integrated it within programs like physician value-based purchasing and accountable care organizations. Much like H-CAHPS for the inpatient setting, the standardized CG-CAHPS survey allows providers and group practices to be compared with each other.[4]

AHRQ developed specific rules to protect the integrity of the survey responses. For example, survey selection is random. Providers are not allowed to influence survey distribution by preventing surveys from being sent to difficult or angry patients. There are also precise guidelines on how the survey is administered, such as by mail or telephone.[5] Questions can be added to the survey, but each survey has a core set of questions that cannot be changed or excluded.[6] The survey assesses various components of care in your clinic. There are also several questions that specifically ask the patient to rate the care delivered by you, the provider.

When scoring the CG-CAHPS survey, the only response that counts is the most favorable response. Depending on which survey your practice uses, patient will either choose from a four-point frequency scale (never, sometimes, usually, always), a six-point frequency scale (where "almost never" and "almost always" are added as response choices), or a three-point expanded yes/no scale (yes, definitely; yes, somewhat; no). On the four and six-point survey, "always" is the most favorable response. On the three-point survey, "yes, definitely" is the most favorable response.[7] As an example, one question on the three-point survey asks, "Did this provider explain things in a way that was easy to understand?" The patient will choose one of the three choices. For most surveys, "yes, somewhat" is considered a good answer. However, for this CG-CAHPS survey, the only response that counts is your number of "yes, definitely" responses. You do not get partial credit for any other answer. It is all or nothing. Another example is a question on the CG-CAHPS survey that asks, "Using any number from 0 to 10, where 0 is the worst provider possible and 10 is the best provider possible, what number would you use to rate this provider?" In any other setting, an eight would be a good score. With the CG-CAHPS rating system, the only scores that count are the number of nines and tens you receive. An eight is essentially equivalent to a zero. When the data is published on websites, such as Physician Compare   (http://www.medicare.gov/physiciancompare/),   the public will only see the percent of patients who gave you the most favorable response.[8]

Throughout this book, I have chosen to highlight questions from the adult CG-CAHPS survey. The adult CG-CAHPS survey is not the only CG-CAHPS survey available. There are other CG-CAHPS surveys available, such as pediatric and patient-centered medical home. Similar provider questions appear on all versions of the survey. The CAHPS® brand of surveys has already expanded across multiple settings including the hospital, clinic, home health, nursing homes, and health plans, with more settings planned for the future.[9] Fortunately, the improvement tips in this book are relevant, regardless of your patient population or practice setting.

Before we move on, I want to point out that although this book focuses on the provider, it is difficult to achieve success without your staff's support. In reality, every member of your team must be on the same page. Everyone must make improving the patient experience one of his or her top priorities. Why is this so important? On the adult survey, there are seven questions that specifically relate to the provider. However, your staff's performance directly impacts your scores. You cannot function independently of your staff, and everyone who works in your clinic must have the same goal of improving patient satisfaction. The following example illustrates this point.

Example:
One of the questions on the CG-CAHPS survey asks, "Would you recommend this provider's office to your family and friends?" Read the scenario to see how your staff's behavior impacts your scores.

Ms. Parmer makes an appointment with you to discuss pain in her left shoulder. Upon arriving at your office, she notes that your receptionist is not particularly friendly. Although the receptionist is skillful at her job, she does nothing to show Ms. Parmer that she is happy to see her or to make her feel at ease.

Two weeks later, Ms. Parmer completes her patient satisfaction survey. She answers the question that asks if she would recommend your office to her family and friends. She thinks back to her experience and remembers the unwelcoming receptionist. Just like that, Ms. Parmer chooses not to select the highest possible score.

You may be thinking, *She's upset with the receptionist. That has nothing to do with me.* Unfortunately, that simply is not true. In reality, patients take into account the entire care experience when rating you and your practice. One hostile receptionist can sabotage your best efforts. As the provider, you can do everything within your control to improve the patient experience. If your staff is not on the same page, you will still have trouble improving your scores. This is why it is so crucial for your clinic to function as a unit. Each person who interacts with your patients must make patient satisfaction one of his or her top priorities.

CHAPTER 2

# Quality and Process Improvement

Did you know that patients judge quality quite differently than providers? If I were to ask you the attributes of a high-quality physician, you would say things like "strong clinical knowledge" or "great diagnostic skills." If you ask patients the characteristics of a high-quality physician, they will say "one who listens to me" or "one who explains things in a way I understand." A 2004 *Wall Street Journal* Online/Harris Interactive poll asked patients what they want from their doctors. The top five responses were: (1) treats you with dignity and respect, (2) listens carefully to your health-care concerns and questions, (3) is easy to talk to, (4) takes your concerns seriously, (5) is willing to spend enough time with me.[10] Do you know what's missing from the top five? Clinical competence, adherence to evidence-based medicine, and an expansive knowledge base, to name a few. Although patients do think these attributes are important, it is difficult for them to differentiate between providers based on these criteria. Patients assume all providers have a basic level of clinical competence. They believe if you graduated from professional school and passed your licensing exams, you are qualified. Thus, patients will distinguish between providers based on an intangible quality: how you make them feel. Do they feel respected by you? Do you listen to them? Do you give them the time they need? Do you seem to care about them as

5

people? This is what matters to patients. How well you demonstrate these intangibles in your practice will determine how your patients rate you. This is why providers must be open to embracing patient satisfaction. Regardless of your clinical expertise, these intangible skills drive satisfaction.

## Sphere of Influence

I want to share another important point before we move on. When I work with providers, I always encourage them to focus on their sphere of control and influence (Figure 1).[11] Doing this will allow you to identify factors within your control. Focusing your energy on things beyond your control is frustrating, time-consuming, and detrimental to progress.

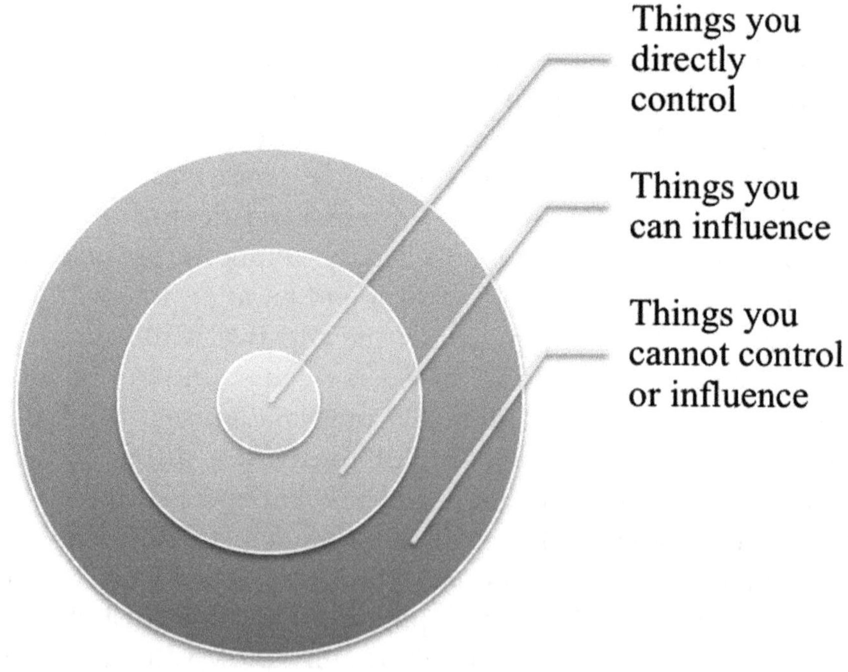


*Figure 1.*

**Things you directly control:** You directly control your actions and behaviors. You chose to read this book, and it is entirely up to you whether you incorporate these techniques into your practice.

**Things you can influence:** You have influence over the members of your staff and their interest in these techniques. You cannot force your staff members to change their attitude or work ethic. However, as a provider and leader in the clinic, you can certainly influence them.

**Things you cannot control or influence:** You cannot control or influence the fact that patient satisfaction surveys exist. Likewise, you have very little control or influence over the survey questions or survey length.

To be successful, you must distinguish between what you can and cannot control. You do not want to waste time or emotional energy on something you cannot change. Refocusing your energy on what you can control will increase your willingness to adopt these techniques and positively impact your patients' experiences. The great news is that all of the suggestions in this book are within your direct control and/or influence. There are no barriers to improvement. All you have to do is commit to the process outlined in this book. As I have seen in my experience working with providers, the process will work if you fully dedicate yourself to improvement.

## Process Improvement

Even if you and your staff agree on the importance of patient satisfaction, you may not achieve your goals without improving your clinic processes and flow. This is where process improvement comes in. It is difficult to focus on patient satisfaction if your clinic is burdened with inefficiency. Process improvement involves taking a critical look at your processes and flow in order to decrease waste and increase value for your patients.[12]

This book is not designed to teach you the fundamentals of process improvement. However, I want to give you an example that demonstrates why process improvement is equally as important as patient satisfaction. It is difficult to have high patient satisfaction without good processes and workflows. Thus, your practice should make process improvement as high a priority as patient satisfaction.

Example: For the past few months, you have noticed yourself running further and further behind. When you first joined the practice, your patients' average wait time was less than five minutes. It is now eighteen minutes. Today, you are running thirty minutes behind for your appointment with Mrs. Myers. Once you finally make it to her room, you apologize for the wait and assure her you will give her the time she needs. You incorporate some of your patient satisfaction tips and ultimately have a wonderful visit with her. She thanks you for your time, and you again apologize for her wait.

As you reflect on the visit, you are frustrated by your wait times. You think about possible reasons, and several come to mind:
* Your clinic is disorganized.
* You recently implemented a new electronic medical record system that decreases efficiency.
* Your clinic layout encourages wasted time.

You know you must do something to address your timeliness. You fear that at some point, your patients will leave your practice if long wait times remain the norm.

In this example, even though the provider uses patient satisfaction techniques, the issues within the clinic's basic processes decrease the impact of these techniques. This clinic should focus on process improvement in addition to patient satisfaction. Until processes improve, long wait times will continue to undermine patient satisfaction efforts. At some point, service recovery efforts will not be enough. Patients will begin leaving the practice, and when that happens, no amount of customer service techniques will bring them back.

# CHAPTER 3

# CG-CAHPS Improvement Tips

Now let us discuss the seven CG-CAHPS provider-specific questions in more detail. As previously stated, these seven questions come from the adult CG-CAHPS survey. Depending on the version you use, it either asks patients to reflect on the care they received from you over the last twelve months or the care they received during their most recent visit.[13] If you use the pediatric survey, it also asks the respondent to reflect on the care the child received.[14]

1. Did this provider explain things in a way that was easy to understand?
2. Did this provider listen carefully to you?
3. Did this provider give you easy-to-understand information about these health questions or concerns?
4. Did this provider seem to know the important information about your medical history?
5. Did this provider show respect for what you had to say?
6. Did this provider spend enough time with you?
7. Using any number from 0 to 10, where 0 is the worst provider possible and 10 is the best provider possible, what number would you use to rate this provider?

**Question 1: Did this provider explain things in a way that was easy to understand?**

Because patients assume all health-care providers have similar levels of competence, they will look for other distinguishing factors when choosing a provider. One of these factors is your ability to communicate and simplify complex concepts. Even though medicine is easy for you, it is confusing for most of your patients. The Internet frequently makes things worse. How many times have you had patients come to your office in a panic after incorrectly diagnosing themselves via the Internet? What patients most need from us is to explain their diagnoses and treatments in ways that are easy for them to understand.

If you struggle in this area, here are five tips for improvement:

1. **Avoid medical lingo.**
   - This is tough to do because medical lingo is a part of who we are as providers. It is engrained in our vocabulary. We are so accustomed to using medical terminology that we are oblivious to it when it slips out in front of the patient.
   - Look at your patient when you are talking, and observe visual cues. If the patient looks confused, he or she probably is. Restate your point while making an extra effort to say it as simply as possible. As you speak, focus on what you are saying, and consciously remind yourself to avoid medical jargon.

2. **Utilize the "teach-back" method to facilitate patient understanding.**
   - "Teach-back" is a method that tests your patient's understanding. You explain your diagnosis and treatment plan to the patient. You then ask the patient to say it back to you in his or her own words.[15]

Example: Start by saying something like, "Mr. Austin, please explain to me, in your own words, how to take your levothyroxine," or, "Mr. Austin, what is your understanding about your diagnosis of hypothyroidism?" Note the difference of these two approaches. With teach-back, you start by querying the patient for his or her understanding. This is different from the way we often practice, in which we provide information to the patient and ask him or her yes or no questions in order to assess understanding.

- If your patient explains it correctly, you affirm his or her understanding. If your patient is unable to explain it correctly, you teach it to him or her again (possibly using different wording). You then ask your patient to state his or her understanding one more time to ensure it is correct.[15]

Example: let's assume Mr. Austin correctly stated the basic information of hypothyroidism that you just spoke of. However, when discussing levothyroxine, he mistakenly said it could be taken in the morning with his breakfast. At this point, you would say something like, "That's great, Mr. Austin. You seem to have a good grasp of what we discussed. The only thing I want to reiterate is how to take your levothyroxine. Food interacts with levothyroxine, so it will not work as well if taken with food. Instead, you should take it first thing in the morning on an empty stomach. As a recap, tell me again your understanding of levothyroxine and how it should be taken."

- For more information, I recommend you review http://www. teachbacktraining.com. This website is filled with great resources on the teach-back method, including videos.[15]

3. **Use diagrams or other visual aids to facilitate your discussion.**
   - Using diagrams and visual aids helps patients conceptualize what you are saying. This can be as simple as drawing a picture on a piece of paper or printing out a diagram. You can use the computer in your room to search for pictures or demonstrate a concept with an app. In the end, it does not matter what format you choose. The important point is that visual aids reinforce the concepts you discussed. Patients are more likely to comply with instructions when they understand them. Diagrams and visual aids facilitate that understanding.

**4. Explain procedures before you do them.**

- Explain the details of the procedure, including the steps you will follow, prior to beginning the procedure. Make sure to discuss how long the procedure will take and what it will feel like.

> Example: "Ms. Sawyer, I'm going to give you a shot of lidocaine to help numb the area. The lidocaine shot will sting, but you will feel better once it starts working. Once the lidocaine kicks in, I'll start the procedure. It should only take a minute."

- While performing the procedure, make sure to communicate with your patient the entire time. Keep the patient informed of how much longer until the procedure is complete. Use encouraging statements, such as, "You're doing great."

> Example: "I'm almost done. I just have one more step to go. You're doing great!"

- Utilize your nurse or medical assistant (MA). A lot of patients find comfort in having someone else in the room to encourage and/or distract them.

> Great idea: Allow your patients to distract themselves by using an electronic device during the procedure. They can listen to music, watch videos, play games, or do anything else that distracts them, as long as it does not interfere with the procedure.

**5. Summarize key points at the end of the visit.**

- During the office visit, you will cover several points in a short amount of time. It is normal for patients to miss important information. One way to address this is to take time to summarize your treatment plan. You can say something like, "In summary…" or, "Let's recap…"

> Example: "Let's summarize what we've talked about today. I'm increasing your lisinopril from 10 mg to 20 mg once a day. You're going to walk at least thirty minutes three times a week, and I'm referring you to a gastroenterologist for your colonoscopy."

**Question 2: Did this provider listen carefully to you?**

Everyone wants to be listened to, and our patients are no different. They come to us because something is bothering them. They are looking to us for help, and they are hopeful we will be able to provide the help they need. They want us to address their problems, but they also want to feel heard. If two doctors are equally competent, patients will usually choose the one who is the better listener. Thus, feeling heard is a key distinguisher patients use when choosing one doctor over another.

If you struggle in this area, here are six tips for improvement:

## 1. Listen.

- Start the visit by asking the patient the top two or three things he or she would like to accomplish during the visit. Due to time constraints, you may not always have time to address a long list of problems. By clarifying and addressing what your patient most wants to accomplish, you will help your patient feel heard.

> Great idea: Develop a patient agenda form (Appendix A). This form solicits the patient's top concerns. You can have the patient complete the form for you to review prior to entering the room, or you may choose to briefly review it with your patient upon entering. Either way, it helps you organize the visit and address your patient's top concerns.[16] This same concept can be accomplished through your electronic medical record. Your nurse or MA can solicit this information and enter it into the electronic medical record. You can also encourage your patients to complete it online prior to the office visit.

- Listen to what your patient is saying, and try to avoid interruptions, except to clarify. One study discovered that it only takes an average of twenty-three seconds before a doctor interrupts his or her patient. The same study revealed that seventy-six percent of physicians interrupt after the patient has only expressed one concern.[17]

> Great idea: Start the office visit by saying, "Tell me your story." This phrase serves as a reminder that all of our patients have a story to tell and that they deserve our time and attention.

- Show you are listening by using conversation continuers. These include head nods and words like "OK," "go on," and "uh-huh."
- We all have patients that ramble. Due to time constraints, you will have patients you must cut off. In these situations, politely redirect them to focus on their most pressing concerns.

> Example: "I know you have a lot you want to discuss. I think all of your concerns are important, but I want to make sure I can give your most important concerns the time they deserve. Please tell me what you are most concerned about today."

**2. Take notes.**
- Taking notes while the patient is talking demonstrates interest in what he or she is saying. It helps you remain engaged in the conversation, and it makes your patient feel that you are listening.
- While taking notes, position yourself so you face your patient. Focus on the patient as much as possible. Minimize your note writing and the amount of time you spend typing on the computer to keep it from interfering with your personal interaction. Taking notes is a great strategy, but you do not want to become so focused on taking notes that it causes you to ignore the patient.

**3. Only interrupt when necessary.**
- Some interruptions are necessary. You must ask clarifying questions to ensure you understand your patient's story.

You will also occasionally turn away from your patient to review the chart or take notes. Help your patient understand that the interruptions are necessary for you to accurately diagnose and treat him or her. When you let your patient know in advance, and explain why the interruptions are beneficial, he or she is less likely to become frustrated.

> Example: "Ms. Taylor, I want to warn you in advance that I will occasionally interrupt you while you are speaking. It will mainly be to ask clarifying questions. It is important for me to completely understand what you are saying to ensure the treatment I choose is the best treatment for you."

## 4. Summarize.

- After your patient tells you his or her story, summarize to make sure you heard everything correctly.

> Example: "Let me make sure I understand this correctly," or, "let me summarize what you said to make sure I've got it."

- Summarize again at the end of the visit, and confirm the care plan. Refer back to the two or three things the patient said he or she wanted to accomplish during the visit. Highlight the goals for the visit, and summarize your plan for each one.

> Example: "Let's recap. The two things you wanted to accomplish today are improving your blood pressure and blood sugar. To help with your blood pressure, I have increased your carvedilol from 3.125 mg to 6.25 mg twice a day. To improve your blood sugars, I have increased your metformin from 500 mg to 1,000 mg twice a day."

**5. Pay attention to nonverbal cues.**

- You can usually tell how your patient is feeling by observing nonverbal cues. Throughout the visit, watch your patient to see if he or she appears scared, anxious, nervous, or sad. Is the patient fidgeting? Does he or she seem about to cry? Does he or she appear ashamed? Does the patient seem as if he or she is holding back? Whenever you pick up on one of these cues, take time to acknowledge it. Address it with your patient, and probe deeper to see what his or her underlying concern is.

> Example: "Mr. Calloway, I can tell something is bothering you. Why don't we discuss it? Tell me about your concerns."

**6. Do not be afraid to use silence.**

- As providers, we are always in a hurry. We inadvertently interrupt our patients and project our thoughts onto them instead of letting them explain themselves. One technique you can use to prevent yourself from interrupting so quickly is selective silence. When there are lulls in the conversation, give your patients at least five seconds to resume their thoughts before jumping in. Patients often hesitate because they are about to reveal something that is difficult for them to discuss. Silence gives them permission to speak, and if you immediately start talking the moment they stop, the opportunity passes.

**Question 3: Did this provider give you easy-to-understand information about your health questions or concerns?**

We all want our patients to follow our instructions. This is why it is so important to make sure they understand what we say. The more our patients understand our instructions and the rationale behind them, the more likely they are to comply. Health care is confusing for patients, and being sick is a stressful experience. Many of our patients are not at their best when we see them in the office. Taking time to clearly explain things and ensuring understanding is invaluable.

If you struggle in this area, here are four tips for improvement.

1. **Use language patients can understand.**
   - In general, avoid using medical terminology. There are, however, a few times when you will want to use medical jargon to ensure your patient knows the proper term. In these instances, make sure to follow the medical terminology with a patient-friendly explanation.

*Example: "What you have is called cellulitis. Cellulitis is the medical term for an infection of the skin."*

2.  **Provide your patients with information about their medical conditions.**

    - You can provide information in many ways. Verbal communication is the primary way we communicate with patients. It is the foundation of our visit. However, patients like to take something that explains their medical condition home with them. This can be a drawing, handout, brochure, website reference, or suggested app. Patients forget much of what is said during the visit, so providing them with information and suggested references is a great way for them to continue learning about their diagnosis, even after the visit ends.

3.  **Write out important information, including your recommendations.**

    - Write out key points from the visit, and ask your patient to take the list home with them. You can handwrite the information or use your electronic medical record to type specific instructions. These instructions can be about anything, but you primarily want to write information that is important for the patient to remember. This would include medication instructions or things you want your patient to do. You want your patient to be able to refer back to your recommendations, even after he or she leaves. Your patient is unlikely to remember all of your recommendations, so writing them down for future reference increases his or her ability to comply.

> Great idea: Write your instructions on your exam table paper. You are going to throw it away anyway. Your patients will love it because the instructions can be written large enough for them to read. This also gives them something to take home and review with their families.

> Great idea: If you are a surgeon or proceduralist, you can really impress your patients by drawing what you have done during your operation or procedure for them to take home with them. This is often done with cardiac surgery. The cardiac surgeon draws a picture of the heart and bypass grafts on a heart-shaped pillow as a memento for the patient to keep. The surgeon and other members of the care team sign it. Adapt this idea for your specialty. Your patients will love it! It's educational, and it provides them with a reminder of the great work you have done.

4. **Find ways to incorporate technology into your practice.**
   - Technology changes rapidly, so recommending a specific service, medical product, or health-care app is not helpful, as new solutions are created every day. As the provider, you should look for ways to leverage technology to make your life and your patients' lives easier. The current generation of patients is less willing to spend its time on things that do not add value. These patients do not want to spend time manually completing paperwork or sitting in a waiting room. They want personalized care that occurs at the time they need it. As patients become more technologically savvy, they expect their health-care provider to incorporate technology into the office practice. Patients want health care to be collaborative, and they view technology as a way to increase their participation in health-care decisions.[18]
   - Here are a few examples of ways you can utilize technology to improve your patient satisfaction. This list will only continue to grow, so it is important for you to occasionally research new technological solutions to see which ones you can adopt in your practice.

✓ Websites and apps that allow patients to securely store and distribute their personal health and insurance information to their provider
✓ Portals that allow patients to communicate with their providers through secure e-mail or messaging systems
✓ Telemedicine and video chats that allow providers to conduct appointments with their patients
✓ Appointment scheduling apps and wait-time notifications
✓ Apps designed to assist with medication management and compatibility assessments
✓ Apps that allow for management of chronic conditions
✓ Apps that improve compliance with the medical regimen by providing reminder alerts
✓ Apps designed to monitor, test, diagnose, and treat
✓ Apps that educate and instruct
✓ Systems that allow providers to share health information and instructions, with the patients' consent, to designated caregivers

**Question 4: How often did this provider seem to know the important information about your medical history?**

Imagine being a patient. Think of how frustrated you would be if you went to see your provider and he or she did not remember basic facts about you or what you discussed during the last visit. Even if you have a great relationship with that provider, you would be frustrated by his or her lack of preparation. Preparation is a key component for achieving success with this question. Even when you have been seeing the same patient for years, you should prepare for the visit each and every time.

If you struggle with this area, here are four tips for improvement.

1. **Review the chart prior to entering the room.**
   - Assuming the records are available, this step is a necessity. Reviewing the chart reminds you of what happened during the last visit and your prior treatment plan.
   - When is the ideal time to do this? You should experiment with various options to decide what works for you. Some providers review all of the next day's patients the evening before. Others review their morning patients before clinic starts and their afternoon patients during lunch. Another method is to review each chart immediately prior to the visit.
   - If you are seeing a new patient and do not have access to his or her chart, use your nurse or medical assistant to solicit pertinent information from the patient. At a minimum, your staff can obtain the patient's chief complaint.
   - Consider using the patient agenda form (Appendix A) to solicit the patient's top concerns. Alternatively, have your staff put the patient's top concerns in the electronic medical record for you to review prior to entering the room.

2. **Specifically reference the chart.**
   - It is not enough to review the chart. You must also refer to the chart *in front of the patient* so that he or she knows you have reviewed it. This helps the patient gain confidence in your knowledge of his or her medical history.

Example: "Ms. Chavez, I was reviewing your chart, and I noticed you were hospitalized three times last year for your emphysema."

> Great idea: Write personal notes about the patient in your chart, and refer to them on subsequent visits. Your patients will be surprised that you remembered and honored that you cared enough to ask. For example, if your patient tells you he or she is about to go on vacation, make a note of this, and ask him or her about it during the next visit.

3. **If you are a specialist, reference why the PCP sent the patient to you and your knowledge of the care plan up to that point.**

   - If you are a specialist, patients often arrive at your office without records. This puts you in a difficult position because you are starting from scratch, yet the patient assumes you have already reviewed their chart. In these situations, acknowledge your patient's potential frustration, but script your response in a positive way. Avoid saying, "I'm sorry I have to ask you so many questions. I requested the records, but they never showed up." Instead, script it more positively, and say something like, "I'm sorry I have to ask you so many questions. As your specialist, I want to know as much as I can about you so that I can create the best treatment plan for you."

4. **Pay attention to your patient's social history.**

   - Knowing a patient's medical history also includes knowing his or her social history. The social history is frequently treated as an afterthought, but from the patient's perspective, it comprises some of the most important facts of his or her life. Taking time to learn about your patient's background, living situation, support system, and barriers to treatment allows you to more thoroughly care for him or her. For example, if you know your patient's only transportation is a shuttle service that runs Monday, Wednesday, and Friday, you will avoid scheduling appointments for Tuesdays and Thursdays, as it would not be possible for him or her to make it. If your patient depends on his or her children to help with medical care, you will schedule appointment times that are also convenient for his or her children. Not learning or acknowledging your patient's social history places you at a disadvantage. You can never fully take care of your patient without understanding his or her social situation. The social situation affects every aspect of your patient's life, including his or her health and ability to comply.[19]

## Question 5: Did this provider show respect for what you had to say?

I think this question is difficult, because we all feel we respect our patients. The key to this question is figuring out how to make it obvious to your patients so they recognize it. Feeling respected is another one of those key factors patients use to help them distinguish one provider from another. Being sick is scary, and many patients are intimidated by the health-care experience. Showing respect is a guaranteed way to create loyalty among your patients.

If you struggle with this area, here are five tips for improvement.

1. **Treat every concern as if it is important.**
   - We all have patients who spend a lot of time telling us their story. This can be frustrating when we know their input will not change the treatment plan. Despite this, allowing patients to tell their story and acknowledging their concerns makes them feel respected. The concerns are obviously important to them, or they would not have bothered to tell you. Let patients know that you are interested in what they are saying and that you have time for them.

**2. Look directly at the patient while he or she is talking, and minimize the amount of time you turn away from the patient.**

- This is much harder to do with the infiltration of computers and electronic medical records in the office. Try these four strategies to counteract the awkwardness of using the computer in the room.
  - Ask your nurse to seat your patients so they are close to you. Do not seat the patient on the exam table if this causes you to turn your back to your patient when using the computer. Place your patient next to you, where you can look at him or her frequently, and only use the exam table for the actual exam.
  - Explain to your patient that you will occasionally turn away from him or her to use the computer during the visit. Patients are more understanding when they know what to expect.
  - Explain what is in it for the patient. Let your patient know his or her records are in the computer and that it helps you to have access to the computer and the records throughout the visit. Say something like, "I will occasionally access your chart during the visit because I want to make sure I accurately capture what you say," or, "I will give you a handout summarizing what we discussed today at the end of the visit. In order to do that, I will occasionally use the computer during our visit." You can figure out what scripting works best for you. The main point is to help your patient understand how turning your attention to the computer from time to time benefits him or her.
  - Use the computer as little as possible while in the room. Complete the nonessential computer tasks before the patient arrives or after the patient leaves.

3. **When possible, involve the patient in the decision-making process and acknowledge his or her input.**
   - As you go through your differential, present various options to your patient, along with the pros and cons of each option. Tell your patient your professional opinion, but when possible, try to make it collaborative. Ask questions like, "Does this plan sound reasonable?" or, "What do you think about this plan?" I realize this approach is not always feasible because there are some decisions that can only be made by the provider. I recommend you look for a few opportunities during each visit to gain input from your patient. Even if it is only once or twice, your patient will be impressed that you respected him or her enough to solicit his or her opinion.
   - In those instances when you do involve your patient in the decision-making process, take time to acknowledge his or her valuable input. Your patient will feel honored that you took time to recognize his or her contribution.

Example: "Thanks for your input, Mrs. Roberts. It was so helpful to hear your thoughts, and I think that by working together, we have come up with a great treatment plan."

4. **If your patient looks uncomfortable with the decision, acknowledge it, and find out why he or she is uncomfortable.**
   - Once you understand the source of your patient's anxiety, talk it through together. Try to discover and address the root cause of the patient's concern. As providers, we take a lot of care in devising the most appropriate plan for our patients. Unfortunately, the best treatment plan is futile if the patient does not follow it due to confusion or fear.

Example: "Mr. Jeter, I can tell you have some hesitations about this plan. Tell me about them. What are your concerns?"

**5. Ask for questions before ending the visit.**

- A recommended alternative to the standard "Do you have any questions?" is to ask, "What questions do you have?" "Do you have any questions?" is a closed-ended question. There are only two responses: yes or no. Patients will often say no, even when they have questions, because they do not want to appear uneducated. Asking an open-ended question, such as "What questions do you have?" gives your patients permission to acknowledge their confusion.

**Question 6: Did this provider spend enough time with you?**

Patients value the time they spend with their providers. Some patients travel long distances to see you. Others wait several days for an appointment. In the end, they all arrive with the hope that your knowledge will improve their situation. Given this expectation, there are few things more frustrating to patients than to feel rushed and feel that their providers did not give them adequate time to express their concerns.

If you struggle in this area, here are four tips for improvement.

**1. Sit down during the patient visit.**

- We have all heard this tip since the first day of training. Why? Because a patient perceives that you spend more time with him or her when you sit down.[20]
- Choose to sit at or lower than eye level with your patient.

- Watch your body language: lean forward, avoid leaning back and crossing your arms, avoid sighing or sounding exasperated, look interested in what the patient is saying, and look like you want to be at work.
- Look directly at your patient while he or she is speaking.

2. **Open the interaction with nonmedical conversation before launching into the visit.**
   - This can be about anything, such as the weather, the patient's plans for the weekend, or his or her family. If you struggle to make small talk, create a standard list of conversation starters you can refer to. After doing this long enough, it will become more natural. There is often a lull in the conversation while you are booting up your computer or waiting for things to load. You can fill this awkward space with small talk.
   - This is also a time when you can reference the nonmedical information about the patient that you included in your previous progress note.

> Example: As you boot up your computer, say, "Mr. Lawson, I know you love gardening. Are you planning to work in the yard this weekend?"

3. **Ask open-ended questions.**
   - Providers have a tendency to ask closed-ended questions where the only response is yes or no. This habit is even more pronounced when we are pressed for time. Closed-ended questions prevent patients from fully explaining themselves or offering additional details. Make a conscious effort to ask several open-ended questions throughout the visit. Open-ended questions are those questions that allow patients to freely

express themselves. For example, start your visit by asking, "How are you doing today?" instead of, "You're here to discuss your high blood pressure. Have you been taking your medication?" The first question invites the patient to lead the conversation. The second question assumes that you already know what your patient wants to discuss, and it leaves little room for your patient to raise issues that are important to him or her.

4. **Make sure your patients know that you have time for them.**
   - At the beginning of the visit, let your patients know that you will give them the time they need. This is especially helpful when you are running late. Let them know that even though you are behind, you will still give them their allotted time. Patients are much more forgiving of late starts when they know they will receive their full time with you.
   - When you ask for questions at the end of the visit, let patients know you have time to address their concerns.

> Example: "What questions do you have? I have time," or, "Is there anything else you want to discuss? I have time."

**Question 7: Using any number from 0 to 10, where 0 is the worst provider possible and 10 is the best provider possible, what number would you use to rate this provider?**

This question is tricky because patients take into account their entire experience with you. When answering this question, they often reflect on multiple interactions with you, as opposed to only the most recent visit. Furthermore, patients will also think about the service provided by your entire team. The receptionist, nurse, and lab technician all influence your patients' responses to this question. This is one reason why it is so important to involve your entire clinic in your patient satisfaction efforts.

If you struggle with this question, here are five tips for improvement.

1. **Engage in daily huddles with your staff.**
   - In its most basic format, a "huddle" is a brief meeting where you and your team discuss patient care. Huddles can occur at any time of day, but in a clinic practice, huddling prior to your first patient is most helpful. You will use the huddle to discuss upcoming patients and make sure you and your staff are on the same page. It also provides an opportunity to discover issues prior to the patient arriving. I recommend you keep your huddle to ten minutes or less and that you stand the entire time to promote efficiency.

   > Example: During the morning huddle, you see that you have a patient coming in for a procedure. This is a good time to make sure your procedure supplies are in stock and ready to go. Your efficiency improves because you do not spend time searching for equipment when the patient arrives.

   > Example: During the morning huddle, you see that your 2:40 p.m. appointment is a patient you are starting on insulin. You know this will be a complicated visit, so you and your staff prepare ahead of time so the visit will run smoothly.

   - Once you get in the habit of huddling, your meeting can evolve to include data analysis and discussion with the goal of driving improvement. Your huddle can take place at a board displaying data and graphs. As you huddle, use your data to guide your discussion. Your data helps you see the issues in your clinic and allows you to prioritize your clinic's improvement projects. Even if you are not ready to take on new projects, huddles are a great way for you and your team to make sure you are all on the same page as you begin your day.

> Example: Your team has identified running late as one of your barriers to high patient satisfaction. You decide as a group to start tracking two data points: the time the patient is roomed and the time the provider enters the room. You collect data daily and document it on the huddle board. Each morning during your team huddle, you briefly turn your attention to your timeliness data. You discuss barriers, suggest improvement ideas, and assign responsibilities. You continuously update your data on your huddle board so your team can analyze the effect of your interventions.

## 2. Send new patients a welcome letter.

- A lot of competition exists for patients. One way to foster loyalty with your new patients is to send them a new patient welcome letter. This is a simple act that helps patients feel special. You can choose to handwrite the note, but most providers do not have time for that. You can create a standard typed letter, but I recommend you sign it in your own handwriting and include a personal note at the end. (*It was so nice meeting you today, Mr. Logan. I hope you feel better soon.*) (Appendix B)

> Great idea: Depending on how complex your practice is, you may find it beneficial to implement a new patient welcome packet. This can be given to your patients before or after the initial visit. It would include any information you think your patients should know to successfully navigate your clinic and health system. You can send it electronically to save resources, or you can post it on your clinic's website. You can even use the video feature on your phone to create a welcome video that you send to all new patients.

3. **Thank patients for choosing your practice.**
   - At the end of the visit, shake your patient's hand, and thank him or her for choosing you and your practice. Patients usually have a choice in their health-care provider. When you take the time to thank your patients, you acknowledge that you understand this. Everyone wants to feel appreciated. Patients are no different. Taking a few moments to thank them goes a long way in establishing loyalty.

4. **End your interaction on a positive note.**
   - Ending on a positive note can be as simple as offering your patients a word of encouragement. Tell them they are doing great and that you are proud of the work they have done to reach their health goals.
   - Another way to end on a positive note is to walk your patients to their next destination, assuming it is close to you. For example, if the checkout desk is around the corner, walk them there. Use this time to build rapport with your patients. Thank them for coming, offer an encouraging word, or simply make small talk. They will be impressed that you took the extra time to show you care.

- Keep a callback log (Appendix C), and commit to calling a select group of patients within one to two days of their visit. You may choose to call your sicker patients to see if they are improving. You may call patients who were apprehensive or unsure about the treatment plan. You may choose patients who underwent procedures to ensure they are doing well. You can also use this time to discuss test results and answer questions. Regardless of what you discuss, your patients will be impressed that you took the time to call. You can also use your electronic medical record system to set alerts and callback reminders.

5. **Let patients know that you value their feedback.**
   - It is perfectly acceptable to let your patients know that they may receive a patient satisfaction survey after the visit. Let them know you value their feedback and would appreciate their taking the time to complete the survey. You can even ask your patients if there was anything you or your office could have done to make the visit more enjoyable. What you cannot do is solicit for specific survey responses or use the exact language from the survey when speaking with patients.

Example:

Acceptable: "Thanks for coming in, Mr. Thomas. You may get a survey asking about your visit in the next few weeks. We are always looking for ways to improve, so we would love to hear your feedback."

NOT acceptable (soliciting for specific responses): "Thanks for coming in, Mr. Thomas. In the next few weeks, you may get a survey asking about your visit today. Please give me a nine or ten for the doctor rating, as those are the only responses that count."

NOT acceptable (using exact survey language): "Thanks for coming in, Mr. Thomas. In the next few weeks, you may get a survey asking about your visit today. Did I show respect for what you had to say, and did I spend enough time with you?"

# CHAPTER 4

# Accountable Care Organization CAHPS Questions

Many of you reading this book are part of an Accountable Care Organization (ACO) or will participate in an ACO in the future. According to the Centers for Medicare & Medicaid Services, Accountable Care Organizations are "groups of doctors, hospitals, and other health-care providers who come together voluntarily to give coordinated high-quality care to their Medicare patients." ACOs have adopted a version of the CAHPS® survey as their patient satisfaction evaluation tool. This survey will only be given to ACO participants once a year. [21]

The ACO-CAHPS survey contains the seven previously discussed provider specific questions. Please refer to chapter three for further information on improving the seven provider specific questions. The ACO-CAHPS survey also contains additional questions not found on the CG-CAHPS survey. These questions are designed to more fully assess your office's overall experience. There are a few questions on the ACO-CAHPS survey that I have chosen not to comment on. Instead, I have selected those questions from the ACO-CAHPS survey that I feel are most relevant to the provider. As a framework, I grouped these additional questions into the following categories:

A.  **Starting and stopping medications**
B.  **Instructions for taking medications**
C.  **Discussions about prescription medications**
D.  **Discussions about surgery and procedures**
E.  **Personal health information**
F.  **Wait times**
G. **Appointments**
H.  **Response times**
I.  **Reminders**
J.  **Visit preparation**
K.  **Follow-up**
L.  **Preventive medicine**
M. **Mental health screen**

For most of these questions, patients can choose one of four responses: never, sometimes, usually, or always. The goal is to get as many "always" responses as possible. For the remaining questions, patients simply answer yes or no.[22] This section is organized to show you the various questions on the survey that fall within the aforementioned categories. After each category, I have listed several suggestions to help you improve your overall scores for that particular group of questions.

## A.  Starting and stopping medications

- In the last 6 months, did you and this provider talk about starting or stopping a prescription medicine? (yes/no)
- Did you and this provider talk about the reasons you might want to take a medicine? (yes/no)
- Did you and this provider talk about the reasons you might **not** want to take a medicine? (yes/no)
- When you and this provider talked about starting or stopping a prescription medicine, did this provider ask what you thought was best for you? (yes/no)

- After you and this provider talked about starting or stopping a prescription medicine, did you **start** a prescription medicine? (yes/no)

**Suggestions for improvement:**

- Take a few moments to explain to patients your rationale for starting or stopping a medication, and query the patient to see if they understand your reasoning.
- Ask if your plan to start or stop a medication sounds reasonable to them and if it is a plan they feel they can follow.
- Ask if the plan for starting or stopping a medication is in line with their personal goals for their health.
- Before ending the visit, ask if they have any questions or concerns about the plan to start or stop a prescription medicine.

## B. Instructions for taking medications

- In the last 6 months, how often did this provider give you easy to understand instructions about how to take your medicines? (never/sometimes/usually/always)
- In the last 6 months, other than a prescription, did this provider give you written information or write down information about how to take your medicines? (yes/no)
- Was the written information this provider gave you easy to understand? (yes/no)
- In the last 6 months, did this provider suggest ways to help you remember to take your medicines? (yes/no)

**Suggestions for improvement:**

- These questions focus on all of the medications a patient takes, as opposed to only new medications. Most of our patients take multiple medications, and time constraints do not allow for a detailed discussion about how to take each one. At the very least, I suggest taking time to discuss new medications, those with dangerous side effect profiles (e.g., anticoagulants), and medicines that are often taken incorrectly (e.g., inhalers).

- Use patient-friendly terminology when explaining medications. Avoid medical jargon.
- Write down your instructions for taking medications for the patient to take home with him or her.
- Use scripting. Make it a point to specifically say something like, "Now I want to discuss a few important instructions about your medications."
- Suggest memory aids—such as pillboxes, calendars, reminders, alarms, and apps—to improve your patient's compliance with taking medications.
- If your patient has a responsible family member who helps with his or her care, use this person to help your patient remember to take his or her medication.

## C. Discussions about prescription medications

- In the last 6 months, did you **take any** prescription medicine? (yes/no)
  - o In the last 6 months, how often did you and anyone on your health care team talk about all the prescription medicines you were taking? (never/sometimes/usually/always)
  - o In the last 6 months, did you and anyone on your health care team talk about how much your prescription medicines cost? (yes/no)

**Suggestions for improvement:**

- Perform medication reconciliation with your patients each and every visit.

- Query your patients at each visit to see if they are having any trouble affording their medications.
- Encourage patients to notify you if they are ever unable to fill a prescription due to cost so you can address the issue.
- Keep a list of inexpensive generic medications and prescribe from this list when possible.

## D. Discussions about surgery and procedures

- In the last 6 months, did you and this provider talk about having surgery or any type of procedure? (yes/no)
- Did you and this provider talk about the reasons you might want to have the surgery or procedure? (yes/no)
- Did you and this provider talk about the reasons you might **not** want to have the surgery or procedure? (yes/no)
- When you and this provider talked about having surgery or a procedure, did this provider ask what you thought was best for you? (yes/no)

**Suggestions for improvement:**

- In addition to discussing your plan, it is vital to make sure your patients understand why you think surgery or a procedure is in their best interest. When patients understand the rationale behind our decisions, they are much more likely to agree with our treatment plan.
- Before ending the discussion, ask your patients the following questions: Do they understand your reasoning? Do they understand the alternatives? Do they understand why you feel one course of action is superior to another? Do they understand what is likely to happen if they choose not to have the surgery or procedure? Do they have any questions or concerns about the plan? Is the surgery or procedure in line with their personal goals for their health?

- Many practices have classes or DVDs to help their patients understand the proposed surgery or procedure. Make sure to utilize these resources.
- Even if your practice does not have an official class or video series, many helpful videos, images, and explanations are found online or through apps that can be recommended to your patients. These resources will help your patients better understand what you are proposing. They also increase satisfaction because they allow patients to contribute to the decision-making process.

### E. Personal health information

- In the last 6 months, did you and this provider talk about how much of your personal health information you wanted shared with your family or friends? (yes/no)
- In the last 6 months, did this provider respect your wishes about how much of your personal health information to share with your family or friends? (yes/no)

### Suggestions for improvement:

- Most offices have some sort of intake form for new patients. Questions relating to your patients' preferences for their personal health information should be included on this form.
- For already established patients, query them on their preferences for use of personal health information, and make sure to note their responses in the medical record.
- Ask your patients about the use of their personal health information in a discreet fashion. Patients may feel uncomfortable requesting their personal health information be restricted in front of the person accompanying them to the visit, especially if they want it restricted from that person.

## F.  Wait times

- Wait time includes time spent in the waiting room and exam room. In the last 6 months, how often did you see this provider **within 15 minutes** of your appointment time? (never/sometimes/usually/always)

**Suggestions for improvement:**

- At the beginning of the book, I mentioned that not every issue could be addressed through patient satisfaction and service recovery efforts. Wait times are one of these things. If you chronically run behind, you and your staff should examine your practice and look for areas of inefficiency and waste. You are more likely to achieve a high score for this question if you first focus on streamlining your work flow. Once your processes are smoother, you can shift your focus to implementing patient satisfaction tools.
- One great suggestion is to distract your patients by giving them something to do. Patients are less cognizant of the time spent waiting when occupied by an activity. Some practices have TVs, magazines, or books. You can also have games to keep your patients occupied, or let them browse a computer or tablet. You may choose to have them read about their medical condition, or watch an educational video. All of these activities create a distraction and fill time. When your patients are occupied, they are less likely to focus on the fact that you are a few minutes behind schedule.
- For a great article on waiting times, I recommend you read "The Psychology of Waiting Lines" by David Maister.[23] This article discusses the psychological impact of waiting and ways to alleviate its negative effects.

## G. Appointments

- In the last 6 months, did you phone this provider's office to get an appointment for an illness, injury, or condition that **needed care right away**? (yes/no)
  - In the last 6 months, when you phoned this provider's office to get an appointment for **care you needed right away**, how often did you get an appointment as soon as you needed? (never/sometimes/usually/always)
- In the last 6 months, did you make any appointments for a **check-up or routine care** with this provider?  (yes/no)
  - In the last 6 months, when you made an appointment for a **check-up or routine care** with this provider, how often did you get an appointment as soon as you needed? (never/sometimes/usually/always)

**Suggestions for improvement:**

- Train your staff to effectively triage calls. Patients are unlikely to use medical terminology when explaining their symptoms. Your staff members should familiarize themselves with the various phrases patients use so they can appropriately triage based on urgency.
- Find alternate ways for your patients to schedule appointments, such as online, with text messaging, through the use of social media, or with apps.
- Increase your number of same-day appointments. Allow patients to be seen the same day for urgent care, routine visits, and health maintenance.
- If you are part of a larger health system, offer patients same-day appointments with any available provider in your system, assuming their preferred provider is unavailable.
- Offer nontraditional office hours. Patients frequently need care outside of the standard Monday–Friday, 8:00

a.m.–5:00 p.m. framework. Finding a way to meet this need, other than referring your patients to urgent care or the ER, greatly improves patient satisfaction.

- Consider alternative visit formats such as telephone visits or video chats.

## H. Response times

- In the last 6 months, did you phone this provider's office with a medical question during regular office hours? (yes/no)
  - o In the last 6 months, when you phoned this provider's office during regular office hours, how often did you get an answer to your medical question that same day? (never/sometimes/usually/always)
- In the last 6 months, did you phone this provider's office with a medical question **after** regular office hours? (yes/no)
  - o In the last 6 months, when you phoned this provider's office **after** regular office hours, how often did you get an answer to your medical question as soon as you needed? (never/sometimes/usually/always)

**Suggestions for improvement:**

- Minimize the number of patient calls sent directly to voice mail. Sending calls to voice mail causes some patients to wait several hours before getting a response. You ideally want your nurses to answer calls as they come in. If calls must go to voice mail, have your nurse check them regularly so that he or she can return patient calls throughout the day.
- When appropriate, utilize other forms of communication with patients, such as e-mail, text messaging, and secure messaging through the electronic medical record, which allows patients to send you messages directly.

- Set goals among your team for response time standards, and track your data. Your goal should be to address all patient phone calls that same day, and definitely within twenty-four hours of the initial call time.

## I. Reminders

- Some offices remind patients about tests, treatment, or appointments in between their visits. In the last 6 months, did you get any reminders from this provider's office between visits? (yes/no)
- In the last 6 months, did this provider's office contact you to remind you to **make an appointment** for tests or treatment? (yes/no)

**Suggestions for improvement:**

- Use an appointment reminder system. Assuming you choose this option, there are many companies that provide this service. Research your options before deciding on a system.
- Suggest to your patients that they download an appointment reminder app. You may want to find a preferred app for this and suggest it to your patients. You can even help your patients enter their next appointment time into the app prior to leaving the office.
- Utilize an app or program that syncs with your office scheduling system. Your office may even choose to create its own app. Once appointments are entered into your scheduling system, they are immediately available for patients to see on their mobile devices.
- Always ensure that your patients' contact information (address, e-mail, phone number) is up-to-date.

- Ask patients their preferred method of communication, such as phone, e-mail, and/or text. Record this information, and use your patient's preferred method to remind him or her to make an appointment.

## J. Visit preparation

- When you visited this provider in the last 6 months, how often did he or she have your medical records? (never/ sometimes/usually/always)

**Suggestions for improvement:**

- Have your staff review upcoming appointments and obtain records for new patients prior to their arrival.

- If you do not have access to a patient's medical record via your electronic medical record system, have your staff obtain a medical release form so you can get records prior to the visit.

- Encourage patients to keep a file of tests and study results done outside of your health system. This can also be done electronically. Ask your patients to provide copies or electronic access to your office prior to their visit. If this is not possible, ask your patients to bring hard copies to the visit with them.

- Recommend your patients keep track of important information about their medical history through secure online programs or apps. This way, it will always be at their disposal.

- Call new patients, or send them a welcome letter or video prior to their first visit with you. Use this opportunity to remind them to bring insurance information and outside records. Ask them to complete all required forms prior to their initial visit. Alternatively, post this information online and refer new patients to your website.

## K. Follow-up

- In the last 6 months, did this provider order a blood test, x-ray, or other test for you? (yes/no)
  - In the last 6 months, when this provider ordered a blood test, x-ray, or other test for you, how often did someone from this provider's office follow up to give you those results? (never/sometimes/usually/always)

**Suggestions for improvement:**

- Make sure to keep a callback log (Appendix C) to track the patients needing follow-up phone calls. I recommend calling no later than one to two days after the appointment. If you expect the wait time to be longer than two days, give your patients an approximate time frame for when you will call.
- Send patients their test results. Some providers choose to send a hard copy via mail. When doing so, make sure to either include a letter summarizing the results or write comments on the lab report. For example: "All of your tests are back and look good," or, "Your cholesterol looks great! Keep up the good work."
- You can also use your electronic medical record system to communicate results and comments to patients. Some EMRs even have the ability to automatically release the results to your patients after a predefined time period.
- Make sure your patients know how to reach you if you do not get back with them as planned. We all have the best

intentions for following up with our patients, but in reality, it occasionally slips our mind. Even though your patients may never contact you, they will be more satisfied knowing they can if the need arises.

## L.  Preventive medicine

- Your health care team includes all the doctors, nurses and other people you see for health care. In the last 6 months, did you and anyone on your health care team talk about specific things you could do to prevent illness?(yes/no)
- In the last 6 months, did you and anyone on your health care team talk about a healthy diet and healthy eating habits? (yes/no)
- In the last 6 months, did you and anyone on your health care team talk about the exercise or physical activity you get? (yes/no)
- In the last 6 months, did you and anyone on your health care team talk with you about specific goals for your health? (yes/no)

**Suggestions for improvement:**

- Put your wait times to good use. Provide patients with information about prevention, nutrition, and physical fitness for them to review while they wait for you. This can be written information or in a digital format.
- Include wellness information on your practice webpage or communicate it to your patients through electronic media before or after visits.
- Write down your wellness recommendations for your patient to take home with them. You can even place them on a prescription to help your patient truly perceive your recommendations as a doctor's order.
- When prescribing medications, take a moment to discuss prevention and actions the patient can take to prevent

illness. Most patients dislike taking medications. They may be more receptive to preventive measures if they feel they will reduce their medication burden.

- Query your patients about their personal health goals and what they want to accomplish through their partnership with you.

## M. Mental health screen

- In the last 6 months, did anyone on your health care team ask you if there was a period of time when you felt sad, empty, or depressed? (yes/no)
- In the last 6 months, did you and anyone on your health care team talk about things in your life that worry you or cause you stress? (yes/no)

## Suggestions for improvement:

- Make it part of your nurse or medical assistant's job to screen for depression and anxiety when rooming patients.
- Choose a validated depression and anxiety screening tool, and routinely incorporate it into the patient visit.
- Place posters in your exam and waiting rooms that encourage patients to discuss depression and anxiety with their provider.

CHAPTER 5

# H-CAHPS Explained

The Hospital Consumer Assessment of Healthcare Providers and Systems (H-CAHPS) survey is a standardized survey created by CMS and the Agency for Healthcare Research and Quality. It is used by hospitals throughout America as a way to measure patient satisfaction and the patient experience. Since 2007, qualifying hospitals must use the H-CAHPS survey and publically report their results or lose a portion of their Medicare reimbursement. Because most hospitals use the H-CAPHS survey, patient responses can easily be compared among hospitals.[24] The survey results are publically available for review on the Hospital Compare website (http://www.medicare.gov/hospitalcompare).[25]

The H-CAHPS survey differs from the CG-CAHPS survey in that it only asks three questions about you, the health-care provider.[26] It also differs from CG-CAHPS because patients usually see more than one provider during their hospitalization. Thus, when patients complete the survey, they are reflecting on their collective experience with every provider who treated them throughout the hospitalization. The H-CAHPS survey is sent to a random sample of discharged patients. It is not just limited to Medicare patients, so patients with all insurance types are eligible to receive the survey.24 The following patients are excluded from receiving a survey: patients discharged to hospice, nursing homes,

53

and skilled nursing facilities; court/law enforcement patients; patients with a home address outside of the United States (unless it is a U.S. territory); no-publicity patients (patients who request their admission be kept private and request not to be surveyed); and patients who are excluded because of the rules or regulations of the state in which the hospital is located.27 The H-CAHPS survey is distributed forty-eight hours to six weeks following discharge. At the time of this book's publication, approved methods for distributing the survey include mail, telephone, mail with telephone follow-up, and interactive voice recognition. Hospitals can choose to add additional questions, although there is a core set of questions that must be asked.24

Even though the H-CAHPS survey does not individually identify the provider, all providers caring for the patient should make patient satisfaction a priority. Most of the improvement tips discussed in this book will help you improve your score on either the CG-CAHPS or H-CAHPS survey. You may notice that several of my improvement suggestions for H-CAHPS are the same suggestions discussed for CG-CAHPS. Many improvement techniques are universal and do not change, regardless of whether you practice in the clinic or the hospital. However, the hospital is a unique environment, so this portion of the book gives improvement strategies specific to the inpatient setting.

Note: the following suggestions are written from the patient's perspective. It is important to remember that the patient's family plays an important role in his or her care while the patient is hospitalized and following discharge. Family members are often the people who complete the patient satisfaction survey. Ask your patient which family members or friends are most important to him or her. If your patient gives you permission, involve these people in his or her care as much as possible.

# CHAPTER 6

# H-CAHPS Improvement Tips

There are three questions on the H-CAHPS survey that specifically assess the care patients receive from their doctors.[26]

1. During this hospital stay, how often did doctors treat you with courtesy and respect?
2. During this hospital stay, how often did doctors listen carefully to you?
3. During this hospital stay, how often did doctors explain things in a way you could understand?

**Question 1: During this hospital stay, how often did doctors treat you with courtesy and respect?**

Every patient wants to feel respected. Being hospitalized can be one of the scariest times in a patient's life. Patients must confront fear, uncertainty, and a loss of control. Given the complexity of inpatient medicine, patients usually play a minor role in their own care. In the midst of these difficult moments, patients appreciate a health-care provider who respects them and solicits their opinion. Below are thirteen improvement suggestions to help your patients feel that they are treated with courtesy and respect in the hospital.

1. **Knock before entering the room.**
   - Knocking before entering is a sign of respect. Our patients are anxious to see us, but they are often in unflattering positions when we enter the room. Even though these situations are routine for you, patients often view their hospitalization as frightening, intimidating, and unsettling. For many patients, this is the first time they have been in a situation where they have little to no control over their condition. Knocking before entering is one small way for you to show your patients respect and help them regain a small amount of control.

2. **Introduce yourself, your role in the patient's care, and your expertise.**
   - Hospitalized patients interact with multiple employees throughout their visit. When meeting a patient, take time to introduce yourself, your role in the patient's care, and your expertise. If you are a consultant, reference the physician who consulted you, and explain how your expertise will benefit the patient in this situation. Your patient will appreciate the fact that you took time to explain your role instead of starting the encounter without any introduction.[28]

Example: "Hello, Ms. Scott. My name is Dr. Dorrah. It's so nice to meet you. I am an internal medicine doctor who only works in the hospital. We call ourselves hospitalists. I will be the primary doctor in charge of your care, and I will coordinate with any specialists you need to see. I have been working here for five years, and I plan to take very good care of you while you are here."

3.  **Review the chart prior to entering the room.**
    *   Assuming the records are available, this step is a necessity. If you are meeting the patient for the first time, reviewing the chart helps you to learn about your patient quickly. You can see what recent changes have occurred in the patient's health. You can learn about any prior hospitalizations and what has occurred since the most recent hospitalization. This is especially important to do if you are a hospitalist, as your interaction with patients is usually limited to the hospitalization. Reviewing the chart is a way for you to quickly learn the pertinent events in your patient's past medical history.
    *   If you are a specialist who is consulting on a patient, pay close attention to the events that have occurred throughout the hospitalization as you review the chart. Every provider who enters the room asks the patient to tell his or her story. From the patient's perspective, this is frustrating because it appears as if the provider did not care enough to learn anything about them before entering the room. Even though you must take your own medical history, I recommend occasionally referencing what you read in the chart. This is a sign of respect, and it shows the patient that you care enough about them to learn their basic history.

4.  **Specifically reference the chart.**
    *   It is not enough to review the chart. You must also refer to the chart *in front of the patient* so he or she knows you have reviewed it. This helps your patient gain confidence in your knowledge of his or her medical history. This is a critical step for hospitalists because the patient knows you do not know him or her as well as his or her primary care physician. You must establish a relationship and build trust with your patient in a short amount of time. Demonstrating

your familiarity with his or her past medical history is one way to do this.

Example: "Ms. Chavez, I reviewed your chart, and I saw that you were also hospitalized last year for shortness of breath. At that time, you were diagnosed with pneumonia."

## 5. Pay attention to your patient's social history.

- A patient's social history is frequently viewed as an afterthought, but from the patient's perspective, it comprises some of the most important facts about his or her life. Taking time to learn about your patient's background, living situation, support system, and barriers to treatment allows you to more effectively care for him or her. You can never fully take care of your patient without understanding his or her social situation, which affects every aspect of your patient's life, including his or her health and ability to comply.[19] For example, if you know your patient has a limited income, you would avoid prescribing expensive name-brand drugs. Instead, you would look for generic alternatives that are more affordable.

## 6. Treat every concern as if it is important.

- We all have patients who spend a lot of time telling us their story. This can be frustrating when we know their input will not change the treatment plan. Despite this, allowing patients to tell their story and acknowledging their concerns makes patients feel respected. The concerns are obviously important to them, or they would not have bothered to mention them. Let patients know that you are interested in what they are saying and that you have time for them.

7.  **Look directly at patients while they are talking.**
    - This is much harder to do with the infiltration of computers and electronic medical records. Many inpatient providers now use computers in the rooms, computers on wheels, or portable tablets when making rounds. This introduces a barrier, as computers draw your attention away from your patient. Try these three strategies to counteract the awkwardness of using a computer or tablet in the room.
        - Tell your patients that you will occasionally turn away to use the computer and explain how it benefits them. For example, let them know that the computer allows you to immediately write orders, and it gives you instant access to their medical records, labs, and radiology reports. Patients are much more understanding when they know what to expect and how it will improve their care.
        - Position the computer so that you are still facing the patient. Make every attempt not to turn your back to your patient when using the computer. If you do turn away, make it as brief as possible.
        - Use the computer as little as possible while in the room. Only use it to complete tasks that are of immediate benefit to your patient. Complete all other tasks outside of the patient room. For example, you may choose to use the computer to show patients their X-rays or enter an order for something your patient requested. These are tasks that patients value. On the other hand, patients do not understand the value of typing a daily progress note. This is an example of something that should be completed outside of the room.

8. **Ask for permission before examining your patients.**
   - Even though your patients come to you for help, they still appreciate being treated in a courteous and respectful manner. One easy way to show respect for your patients is to ask their permission before beginning the physical exam.[28]

9. **When possible, involve the patient in the decision-making process and acknowledge his or her input.**
   - Throughout the hospitalization, look for opportunities to gain input from your patient. I realize this approach is not always feasible because hospital medicine is complex. There are many decisions that can only be made by the provider. However, if more than one treatment option is acceptable, try to engage your patient in collaborative decision making. Present the options, along with your professional opinion, and ask the patient what he or she thinks. Ask if the care plan sounds reasonable or if the patient has any concerns. Your patient will appreciate that you respected him or her enough to solicit his or her opinion.
   - When you do involve your patient in the decision-making process, make sure you acknowledge his or her contribution. Your patient will feel honored that you took a moment to recognize his or her input.

Example: "Thanks for your input, Mrs. Roberts. It was so helpful to hear your thoughts, and I think that together, we have come up with a great treatment plan."

10. **If the patient looks uncomfortable with the decision, acknowledge it and find out why he or she is uncomfortable.**
    - Once you understand the source of your patient's anxiety, talk it through together. Try to discover and address the root cause of your patient's concern. As providers, we put a lot of effort into devising the most appropriate care plan. Unfortunately, the best treatment plan is futile if the patient does not follow it due to confusion or fear. This is especially important for inpatient providers and hospitalists. Patients are most loyal to their regular physicians. If a patient feels uncomfortable about your treatment plan, he or she often will not follow it or will wait to get permission from his or her primary care provider. Alleviating the patient's concerns prior to discharge helps to avoid additional anxiety and delays in the initiation of your treatment plan.

> Example: "Mr. Jeter, I can tell you have some hesitations about this plan. Tell me about them. What are your concerns?"

11. **Ask for questions before leaving the room.**
    - A recommended alternative to the standard "Do you have any questions?" is to ask, "What questions do you have?" "Do you have any questions?" is a closed-ended question. There are only two responses: yes or no. Patients will often say no, even when they have questions, because they do not want to appear uneducated. Asking an open-ended question such as, "What questions do you have?" gives your patients permission to acknowledge their confusion.

**12. End each interaction on a positive note.**

- Ending on a positive note can be as simple as offering your patients a word of encouragement or telling them it was good to see them and that you will talk again soon. You could also take a moment to ask your patients if they need anything. Being hospitalized is frustrating, and your patients will appreciate any small gesture of kindness.

**13. End the hospitalization on a positive note.**

- At the end of the hospitalization, take a moment to thank your patients for choosing your health-care facility. With the exception of a medical emergency, most hospitalized patients have a choice in where they are admitted. Everyone wants to feel appreciated, and patients are no different. Taking a few moments to thank them goes a long way in establishing loyalty.
- Let patients know you value their feedback.
  - o It is perfectly acceptable to let your patients know that they may receive a patient satisfaction survey after their hospitalization. Let them know that you value their feedback and appreciate their taking the time to complete the survey. You can even ask your patients if there was anything you or the staff could have done to make the visit more enjoyable. Even if you cannot personally fix the issues, you can refer their suggestions to the appropriate person. Please remember that you cannot solicit for specific survey responses or use the exact language from the survey when speaking with patients.

Example:

Acceptable: "It was very nice to meet you, Mr. Thomas. You may get a survey asking about your hospitalization in the next few days. We are always looking for ways to improve, so we would love to hear your feedback."

NOT acceptable (soliciting for specific responses): "It was very nice to meet you, Mr. Thomas. You may get a survey asking about your hospitalization in the next few days. Our hospital administration pays close attention to those surveys, so please rank us with "always" on the survey questions."

NOT acceptable (using exact survey language): "It was very nice to meet you, Mr. Thomas. You may get a survey asking about your hospitalization in the next few days. Did I always treat you with courtesy and respect, listen to you, and explain things in a way you could understand?"

## Question 2: During this hospital stay, how often did doctors listen carefully to you?

Everyone wants to be listened to, and our patients are no different. They are hospitalized because something is bothering them, and they are looking to us for help. In addition to addressing their problems, our patients want to feel heard. The hospital is a frustrating environment. Oftentimes, patients just want someone who will listen to them. As providers, we cannot always cure our patients' illnesses, but we can always take a moment to listen. Below are nine improvement suggestions to help your patients feel that you listened carefully to them.

1.  **Listen.**
    - More than anything, patients want to feel heard. They want providers who take the time to listen to them. Try to avoid interruptions, except to clarify. One study discovered it only takes an average of twenty-three seconds before a doctor interrupts his or her patient. The same study revealed that seventy-six percent of physicians interrupt after the patient has only expressed one concern.[17]
    - Inpatient providers and hospitalists are often under strict time constraints. You frequently do not have time to address a long list of problems. In these instances, it is OK to politely redirect your patient back to his or her most pressing medical issue. Another strategy is to set boundaries regarding what issues must be addressed while hospitalized and what issues can be deferred to the outpatient setting. Spend your time on the most urgent issues. Only address less critical issues as time permits. Make sure you explain to your patient why you view some issues to be more important than others, as every issue is important to your patient. Finally, if you discover that there is one issue the patient wants to address above all others, decide whether this is something that can reasonably be addressed as an inpatient. Addressing his or her chief concern, even if you find it trivial, is one way to guarantee your patient feels heard.

Example: "I know you have a lot you want to discuss, Mr. Turner. You were admitted to the hospital with chest pain, so this is the most important thing we must address while you are here. I can tell you are also quite concerned about your foot pain. Because it is so bothersome for you, I will look into this further. My top priority, however, will still be evaluating your chest pain."

> Great idea: Create a way for patients to record their questions for the doctor so they will not forget. Family members can also write down questions, as they often are not present during rounds. This can involve something as simple as a sheet of paper, a small notepad, a white board, or a secure online portal.

- When speaking with patients, show you are listening by using conversation continuers. These include head nods and words like, "OK," "go on," and "uh-huh."

2. **Take notes.**
   - This suggestion is most applicable for the initial history and physical or when doing a consult. Taking notes while the patient is talking demonstrates interest in what he or she is saying. It helps you remain engaged in the conversation, and it makes your patient feel that you are listening.
   - While taking notes, position yourself so you face your patient. This allows you to focus on mphe patient as much as possible. Minimize your note writing and the amount of time you spend typing on the computer to keep it from interfering with your personal interaction. Taking notes is

a great strategy, but you do not want to become so focused on taking notes that it causes you to ignore the patient.

3. **Only interrupt when necessary.**
   - Some interruptions are necessary. For example, you may have to interrupt to ask clarifying questions to ensure you understand your patient's story. Warn your patients before beginning that you may occasionally interrupt them. When you let them know in advance and explain why you must occasionally interrupt, your patients are less likely to become frustrated.

   > Example: "Ms. Taylor, I want to warn you in advance that I will occasionally interrupt you while you are speaking. It will mainly be to ask clarifying questions. It is important for me to completely understand what you are saying to ensure the treatment I choose is the best one for you."

4. **Summarize key points of the patient's story and your treatment plan.**
   - When doing an initial history and physical or consult, take a moment to summarize the key points after the patient finishes telling you his or her story. This will give you a chance to ensure you understood the patient correctly. On follow-up rounding days, you can still summarize the main issues raised by the patient that day.

   > Example: "Let me make sure I understand this correctly," or, "let me summarize what you said to make sure I've got it."

- Summarize your treatment plan. Providers cover a lot of information during each interaction, so taking a moment to summarize the daily treatment plan before you leave the room is helpful.

> Example: "Let's recap. Your blood pressure has been running high, so I'm going to increase your carvedilol from 3.125 mg to 6.25 mg twice a day. To improve your blood sugars, I have increased your insulin from 10 units to 12 units at bedtime."

5. **Pay attention to nonverbal cues.**
   - You can usually tell how your patient is feeling by observing nonverbal cues. During each interaction, watch your patient to see if he or she appears scared, anxious, nervous, or sad. Whenever you pick up on one of these clues, take time to acknowledge it. Address it with your patient and probe deeper to see what his or her underlying concern is.

> Example: "Mr. Calloway, I can tell something is bothering you. Why don't we discuss it? Tell me about your concerns."

6. **Do not be afraid to use silence.**
   - As providers, we are always in a hurry. We inadvertently interrupt our patients and project our thoughts onto them instead of letting them explain themselves. One technique you can use to prevent yourself from interrupting so quickly is selective silence. When there are lulls in the conversation,

give your patients at least five seconds to resume their thoughts before jumping in. Patients often hesitate because they are about to reveal something that is difficult for them to discuss. Silence gives them permission to speak, and if you immediately start talking the moment they stop, the opportunity passes.

7.  **Consider sitting down during the patient visit.**
    *   When you sit down, patients perceive that you spend more time with them.[19] This perception of having received quality time makes them feel listened to. Choose to sit at or lower than eye level with your patient. You can request permission to sit on the edge of the bed, in a chair, or on a couch in the room.

    *   Watch your body language. Lean forward, avoid sighing or sounding exasperated, look interested in what the patient is saying, avoid leaning back and crossing your arms, and look like you want to be at work.

    *   Look directly at your patient while he or she is speaking. Avoid the temptation to spend most of your time looking at the computer or your notes.

8.  **Ask open-ended questions.**
    *   Providers have a tendency to ask closed-ended questions where the only response is yes or no. This habit is even more pronounced when we are pressed for time. Closed-ended questions prevent the patient from fully explaining themselves or offering additional details. Open-ended questions are those questions that allow patients to freely express themselves. For example, start your daily visit by asking, "How are you doing today?" instead of, "How is your cough?" The first question invites the patient to lead the

conversation. The second question leaves little room for your patient to raise any issues beyond what you want to discuss.

## 9. Make your patients feel that you have time for them.

- Make it a point to let your patients know that you will give them the time they need. You may choose to illustrate this by sitting during the visit. You can also demonstrate this by starting the visit with an open-ended question and limiting your interruptions. At the end of the visit, you should query for questions and let your patients know you have time to address their concerns. Pay attention to your body language. Avoid fidgeting and looking bored. Avoid glancing at the clock or standing with your hand on the door. All of these strategies help your patients to see that although you are busy, you are still willing to take time to listen to them.

## Question 3: During this hospital stay, how often did doctors explain things in a way you could understand?

Most patients do not have any medical training. Even though the Internet has made it easier for patients to educate themselves about their illness or injury, they still rely on their providers' explanations. As providers, we must always seek to explain things in patient-friendly terms. Below are nine improvement suggestions to help your patients feel that you explained things in a way they could understand.

## 1. Avoid medical lingo.

- This is tough to do because medical lingo is a part of who we are as providers. It is engrained in our vocabulary. We are so accustomed to using medical terminology that we are oblivious to it when it slips out in front of the patient.

- One tip that may help is to look at your patient to observe visual cues while you are talking. If the patient looks confused, he or she probably is. Restate your point while making an extra effort to say it as simply as possible. As you speak, focus on what you are saying, and consciously remind yourself to avoid medical jargon.

2. **Explain physical exam findings.**
   - Tell your patients what you find as you perform the physical exam, and explain how this information helps you. Patients often worry that their physical exam is abnormal, and this fear increases if the provider makes comments such as, "Hmmm," during the exam. Let your patients know in patient-friendly terms what you learned from the physical exam and how it influences your treatment decision.

> Example: "When I pressed on the upper right part of your belly, you had quite a bit of pain. I think the abdominal pain you described may be due to your gallbladder. I am going to order an ultrasound to look more closely at your gallbladder to see if you have an infection."

3. **Utilize the "teach-back" method to facilitate patient understanding.**
   - "Teach-back" is a method that tests your patient's understanding. You explain your diagnosis and treatment plan to the patient. You then ask the patient to say it back to you in his or her own words.[15]

> Example: "Mr. Austin, I'm about to discharge you, but I wanted to quickly recap. What is your understanding of your diagnosis of congestive heart failure?"

> Example: "I want to make sure we're on the same page. What would you do with your furosemide if you weigh yourself and notice more than a three-pound weight gain in one day?"

- Note the difference of these two approaches. With teach-back, you start by querying the patient for his or her understanding. This is different from the way we often practice, in which we provide information to the patient and ask him or her yes or no questions in order to assess understanding.[15]
- If your patient explains it correctly, you affirm his or her understanding. If he or she misses a key point, you restate the information in a way the patient can understand. You then ask your patient to state his or her understanding one more time to ensure it is correct.[15]

> Example: let's assume Mr. Austin correctly reviews the basic points of congestive heart failure. However, when discussing the new beta-blocker you prescribed, he becomes confused. You could say something like, "That's great, Mr. Austin. You have a good grasp on what we discussed. The only thing I want to reiterate is how to take your metoprolol. I have prescribed the extended-release pill, so you only have to take it once a day instead of twice." Prior to ending your visit, you would query again by saying, "As a recap, tell me once more your understanding of how to take your metoprolol."

- For more information, I recommend you review http://www.teachbacktraining.com. This website is filled with great resources on the teach-back method, including instructional videos.[15]

4. **Use diagrams or other visual aids to facilitate your discussion.**
   - Using diagrams and visual aids helps the patient conceptualize what you are saying. This can be as simple as drawing a picture on a piece of paper or printing out a diagram. You can use the computer in your room to search for pictures or demonstrate a concept with an app or video. In the end, it does not matter what format you choose. The important point is that visual aids reinforce the concepts you discussed. A patient is more likely to comply with instructions when he or she understands them. Diagrams and visual aids facilitate that understanding.

**5. Explain procedures before you order or perform them.**

- If you are an inpatient provider or hospitalist who performs procedures, explain the details of the procedure, including the steps you will follow prior to starting the procedure. Make sure to discuss how long the procedure will take and what it will feel like.

> Example: "Ms. Sawyer, I'm going to give you a shot of lidocaine to help numb the area. The lidocaine shot will sting, but you will feel better once it starts working. Once the lidocaine kicks in, I'll start the procedure. It should only take a few minutes."

- While performing the procedure, make sure to communicate with the patient the entire time. Keep them informed of how much longer until the procedure is complete. Use encouraging statements such as, "You're doing great."

> Example: "I'm almost done. I just have one more step to go. You're doing great!"

- Utilize your nurse or tech. A lot of patients find comfort in having someone else in the room to encourage and/or distract them.

> Great idea: Allow your patients to distract themselves by using an electronic device during the procedure. They can listen to music, watch videos, play games, or do anything else that distracts them as long as it does not interfere with the procedure.

- Even if you are not personally performing the procedure, you can still give your patient a basic overview of the procedure and why you feel it is necessary.

## 6. Use language the patient can understand.

- In general, avoid using medical terminology. There are, however, a few times when you will want to use medical jargon to ensure your patient knows the proper term. In these instances, make sure to follow-up the medical terminology with a patient-friendly explanation.

> Example: "What you have is called cellulitis. Cellulitis is our medical term for an infection of the skin."

## 7. Provide patients with information about their medical conditions.

- You can provide information in many ways. Verbal communication is the primary way we communicate with patients. However, patients like to have something that explains their medical condition to keep or refer back to. This can be a drawing, handout, DVD or video, website reference, educational tool, or app. Patients forget much of what we tell them, and this is even worse in the inpatient setting, where patients may be very ill, experiencing side effects of medication, or are in pain. Providing hospitalized patients with information is a great way for them to continue learning about their diagnosis once you leave the room and after they are discharged from the hospital.

8. **Write out important information, including your recommendations.**
   - Write out important instructions and recommendations for patients to take home with them. You can handwrite the information or use your electronic medical record to type specific instructions. These instructions can be about anything, but you primarily want to write information that is important for the patients to remember. This would include things like medication or postdischarge instructions. You want your patients to be able to refer back to your recommendations, even after they are discharged. Your patients are unlikely to remember all of your advice, so writing it down for future reference increases their ability to comply.

> Great idea: If you are a surgeon or proceduralist, you can really impress your patients by drawing what you have done during your operation or procedure for them to keep. Alternatively, if you have taken pictures during the procedure (e.g., gastric ulcer seen during endoscopy procedure), give your patients copies of the pictures for their records. It is educational, and it provides them with a reminder of the great work you have done.

9. **Find ways to incorporate technology into your practice.**
   - Technology changes rapidly, so recommending a specific service, medical product, or health-care app is not helpful, as new solutions are created every day. As the provider, you should look for ways to leverage technology to make your

life and your patients' lives easier. Patients want health care that is safe, efficient, effective, timely, and personalized. As patients become more technologically savvy, they expect their health-care providers to use technology to meet these expectations. Finally, patients want health care to be collaborative, and they view technology as a way to increase their participation in health-care decisions.[18]

- Here are a few examples of ways you can utilize technology to improve your patient satisfaction. This list will only continue to grow, so it is important for providers to occasionally research new technological solutions to see which ones can be adopted in their practice.

  ✓ Websites and apps that allow patients to securely store and distribute their personal health and insurance information to their provider
  ✓ Portals that allow patients to communicate with their providers through secure e-mail or messaging systems
  ✓ Telemedicine and video chats that allow providers to conduct appointments with their patients
  ✓ Appointment scheduling apps and wait-time notifications
  ✓ Apps designed to assist with medication management and compatibility assessments
  ✓ Apps that allow for management of chronic conditions
  ✓ Apps that improve compliance with the medical regimen by providing reminder alerts
  ✓ Apps designed to monitor, test, diagnose, and treat
  ✓ Apps that educate and instruct
  ✓ Systems that allow providers to share health information and instructions, with the patients' consent, to designated caregivers

# CHAPTER 7

# Conclusion

Now that you are finished, what do you think? Did you learn anything new? Did you see any tips you can immediately incorporate into your practice? Like most providers, you have probably heard these suggestions before. The key to success is to consistently incorporate these suggestions into your practice. Trust me when I say that I understand you frequently feel overworked. Focusing on patient satisfaction can seem like one more task on your to-do list. My advice is to start small. Do not try to incorporate all of the improvement suggestions at once. Instead, start by choosing three things. Chapters eight and nine outline a condensed list of all of the suggestions presented in this book. Review these lists, and choose three things you can consistently start doing. Consistency is key because the tips will only work if performed regularly. I also recommend starting now! Your first three things should be suggestions you can immediately incorporate into your practice. Write down your improvement strategies, and post them where you can see them every day. Remind yourself of your three tips daily. Once you have improved your first three things, choose three more. I know it can be frustrating, but these tips really do work. Commit to it, stay with it, and don't give up. Good luck!

# CHAPTER 8

# Condensed CG-CAHPS Tips

**A. Did this provider explain things in a way that was easy to understand?**
1. Avoid medical lingo.
2. Utilize the "teach-back" method to facilitate patient understanding.
3. Use diagrams or other visual aids to facilitate your discussion.
4. Explain procedures before you do them.
5. Summarize key points at the end of the visit.

---

**B. Did this provider listen carefully to you?**
1. Listen.
2. Take notes.
3. Only interrupt when necessary.
4. Summarize.
5. Pay attention to nonverbal cues.
6. Do not be afraid to use silence.

---

**C. Did this provider give you easy-to-understand information about your health questions or concerns?**
1. Use language the patient can understand.
2. Provide your patients with information about their medical conditions.
3. Write out important information, including your recommendations.
4. Find ways to incorporate technology into your practice.

---

**D. Did this provider seem to know the important information about your medical history?**
1. Review the chart prior to entering the room.
2. Specifically reference the chart.
3. If you are a specialist, reference why the PCP sent the patient to you and your knowledge of the care plan up to that point.
4. Pay attention to your patient's social history.

---

**E. Did this provider show respect for what you had to say?**
1. Treat every concern as if it is important.
2. Look directly at the patient while he or she is talking, and minimize the amount of time you turn away from the patient.
3. When possible, involve the patient in the decision-making process and acknowledge his or her input.
4. If your patient looks uncomfortable with the decision, acknowledge it and find out why he or she is uncomfortable.
5. Ask for questions before ending the visit.

---

**F. Did this provider spend enough time with you?**
   1. Sit down during the patient visit.
   2. Open the interaction with nonmedical conversation before launching into the visit.
   3. Ask open-ended questions.
   4. Make sure your patients know that you have time for them.

---

**G. Using any number from 0 to 10, where 0 is the worst provider possible and 10 is the best provider possible, what number would you use to rate this provider?**
   1. Engage in daily huddles with your staff.
   2. Send new patients a welcome letter.
   3. Thank patients for choosing your practice.
   4. End your interaction on a positive note.
   5. Let patients know that you value their feedback.

# CHAPTER 9

# Condensed H-CAHPS Tips

**A. During this hospital stay, how often did doctors treat you with courtesy and respect?**
1.  Knock before entering the room.
2.  Introduce yourself, your role in the patient's care, and your expertise.
3.  Review the chart prior to entering the room.
4.  Specifically reference the chart.
5.  Pay attention to your patient's social history.
6.  Treat every concern as if it is important.
7.  Look directly at patients while they are talking.
8.  Ask for permission before examining your patients.
9.  When possible, involve the patient in the decision-making process and acknowledge his or her input.
10. If the patient looks uncomfortable with the decision, acknowledge it and find out why he or she is uncomfortable.
11. Ask for questions before leaving the room.
12. End each interaction on a positive note.
13. End the hospitalization on a positive note.

**B. During this hospital stay, how often did doctors listen carefully to you?**
1. Listen.
2. Take notes.
3. Only interrupt when necessary.
4. Summarize key points of the patient's story and your treatment plan.
5. Pay attention to nonverbal cues.
6. Do not be afraid to use silence.
7. Consider sitting down during the patient visit.
8. Ask open-ended questions.
9. Make your patients feel that you have time for them.

---

**C. During this hospital stay, how often did doctors explain things in a way you could understand?**
1. Avoid medical lingo.
2. Explain physical exam findings.
3. Utilize the "teach-back" method to facilitate patient understanding.
4. Use diagrams or other visual aids to facilitate your discussion.
5. Explain procedures before you order or perform them.
6. Use language the patient can understand.
7. Provide patients with information about their medical conditions.
8. Write out important information, including your recommendations.
9. Find ways to incorporate technology into your practice.

# Appendices

All resources included in these appendices can be found on my website, **www.drtrinadorrah.com**.

## Appendix A—Sample Patient Agenda Form

### The Doctor's Office
Patient Agenda Form

Patient name _________________________________________

Date of visit _________________________________________

What three things do you most want to discuss today?

1. _________________________________________
2. _________________________________________
3. _________________________________________

Do you need any of the following items today?

________Refills

________New prescriptions

________Referrals

________Completions of forms

________Work/school excuse

________ Other (please explain) _________________________

_________________________________________

# Appendix B—Practice Welcome Letter

Dear [patient name],

It is my pleasure to welcome you as a patient to [insert practice name]. We know you have a choice of health-care providers, and we truly appreciate your decision to become our patient. We value our patients, so please let us know if there is ever anything we can do to improve your experience.

At [insert practice name], our goal is to treat every patient with respect, compassion, and professionalism. We have an excellent staff that truly desires to partner with you to improve your health.

Our office is open Monday–Friday, from 8:00–5:00 p.m. Our number is 555-555-5555. If it is after hours, our answering service will assist you. If it is a medical emergency, please call 911.

At [insert practice name], we believe in working together with our patients to help you reach your health-care goals. We will guide and lead you, but by working together, we hope your relationship with [insert practice name] will be one you cherish for many years to come.

Sincerely,
[Doctor's name]

*[Write a personal message in your own handwriting.]*

Ms. Johnson,

It was great meeting you today! I look forward to getting to know you better.

Dr. Dorrah

# Appendix C—Sample Callback Log

| The Doctor's Office Callback Log | | | | | | |
|---|---|---|---|---|---|---|
| Patient name | Medical record number | Date of visit | Chief complaint | Reason for callback | Date of callback | Completed (yes/no) |
| Smith, Sue | 2121211 | March 15 | Pneumonia | Inquire about improvement | March 17 | ✔ |
| | | | | | | |
| | | | | | | |
| | | | | | | |
| | | | | | | |
| | | | | | | |
| | | | | | | |
| | | | | | | |
| | | | | | | |
| | | | | | | |
| | | | | | | |
| | | | | | | |
| | | | | | | |
| | | | | | | |

## Appendix D—Wait Time Apology Letter

### The Doctor's Office

Dear [patient name],

I wanted to personally apologize for your wait today. At [insert practice name], we always strive to see our patients in a timely fashion. Unfortunately, that did not happen for you today, and I just wanted to let you know that I am sorry for the inconvenience. Please know that we are always working to improve. Reducing wait times for our patients is always one of our top priorities. Thank you again for your patience, and I look forward to seeing you at your next visit.

Sincerely,
[Doctor's name]

*[Write a personal message in your own handwriting.]*

Ms. Johnson,

It was great seeing you today. I apologize for your wait.

Dr. Dorrah

# References


1. Hulya Aksu, "Customer Service: the New Proactive Marketing," *Huffington Post*, March 26, 2013, http://www.huffingtonpost.com/hulya-aksu/customer-service-the-new-_b_2827889.html.

2. Dale Shaller, "CGCAHPS: What Physician Groups Need to Know," *Association for Patient Experience*, last modified April 5, 2012, http://www.patient-experience.org/Education-Research/Article-Archive/CGCAHPS--Why-These-Should-be-on-Your-Radar.aspx.

3. "Value-Based Payment Modifier," Centers for Medicare & Medicaid Services, last modified August 8, 2013, http://www.cms.gov/Medicare/Medicare-Fee-for-Service-Payment/PhysicianFeedbackProgram/ValueBasedPaymentModifier.html.

4. "Frequently Asked Questions About CGCAHPS," *Press Ganey Associates*, accessed October 6, 2013, http://www.pressganey.com/researchResources/governmentInitiatives/CGCAHPS/faqs.aspx.

5. "Fielding the CAHPS Clinician & Group Surveys," *Agency for Healthcare Research and Quality*, last modified September 1, 2011, https://cahps.ahrq.gov/surveys-guidance/docs/1033_CG_Fielding_the_Survey.pdf.

6. "Preparing a Questionnaire Using the CAHPS Clinician & Group Surveys," *Agency for Healthcare Research and Quality*, last modified September 1, 2011, https://cahps.ahrq.gov/surveys-guidance/docs/1032_cg_preparing_a_questionnaire.pdf.

7. "CAHPS Clinician & Group Surveys: Overview of the Questionnaires," *Agency for Healthcare Research and Quality*, last modified June 15, 2012, https://cahps.ahrq.gov/surveys-guidance/docs/2350_cg_overview_of_questionnaires.pdf.

8. "An Introduction to CGCAHPS," *Studer Group*, accessed October 30, 2013, https://www.studergroup.com/our-impact/an-introduction-to-cg-cahps.

9. Jodie Cunningham, "Preparing for Future CAHPS Measurement," *Press Ganey Associates*, last modified April 15, 2013, http://www.pressganey.com/Libraries/2013_Regionals_Presentations/Preparing_for_Future_CAHPS_Measurement.sflb.ashx.

10. Beckey Bright, "Doctors' Interpersonal Skills Valued More Than Their Training or Being Up-to-Date," *Harris Interactive Poll, The Wall Street Journal Online* 3, no. 19, September 28, 2004, http://online.wsj.com/article/SB109630288893728881.html.

11. Stephen R. Covey, *The 7 Habits of Highly Effective People*. New York: Free Press, 2004.

12. Donald M. Berwick and Andrew D. Hackbarth, "Eliminating Waste in US Health Care," *JAMA* 307, no. 14 (April 11, 2012): 1513–6.

13. Centers for Medicare & Medicaid Services, "CAHPS® Clinician & Group Surveys: Adult 12-month questionnaire 2.0," accessed July 19, 2013, https://cahps.ahrq.gov/clinician_group/cgsurvey/adult12mocoresurveyeng2.pdf.

14. Centers for Medicare & Medicaid Services, "CAHPS® Clinician & Group Surveys: Child 12-month questionnaire 2.0," accessed October 10, 2013, https://cahps.ahrq.gov/clinician_group/cgsurvey/child12mocoresurveyeng2.pdf.

15. "10 Elements of Competence for Using Teach-Back Effectively," *Always Use Teach-back! training toolkit*, accessed June 22, 2013, http://www.teachbacktraining.com.

16. Ronald M. Epstein, Larry Mauksch, Jennifer Carroll, and Carlos Roberto Jaén, "Have You Really Addressed Your Patient's Concerns?" *Family Practice Management* 15, no. 3 (March 2008): 35–40, http://www.aafp.org/fpm/2008/0300/p35.html.

17. M. Kim Marvel, Ronald M. Epstein, Kristine Flowers, and Howard B. Beckman, "Soliciting the Patient's Agenda: Have We Improved?" *Journal of the American Medical Association* 281 (January 20, 1999): 283–287, doi:10.1001/jama.281.3.283.

18. Dan Gonos and Wei-Nchih Lee, "Healthcare on the Move: Leveraging Mobile Technologies to Deliver Personalized, Patient-Centric Healthcare," Viewpoint paper, Hewlett-Packard Development Company, last modified April 2013, http://h20195.www2.hp.com/v2/GetPDF. aspx%2F4AA4-5855ENW.pdf.

19. Frederic W. Platt and Geoffrey H Gordon, *Field Guide to the Difficult Patient Interview.* Philadelphia: Lippincott Williams & Wilkins, 2004.

20. K. J. Swayden, K. K. Anderson, L. M. Connelly, J. S. Moran, J. K. McMahon, and P. M. Arnold, "Effect of Sitting vs. Standing on Perception of Provider Time at Bedside: A Pilot Study," *Patient Education and Counseling* 86, no. 2 (February 2012): 166–71, doi: 10.1016/j. pec.2011.05.024.

21. Centers for Medicare & Medicaid Services, "Accountable Care Organizations (ACO)," last modified March 22, 2013, http://www.cms.gov/Medicare/Medicare-Fee-for-Service-Payment/ ACO/index.html?redirect=/aco.

22. Centers for Medicare & Medicaid Services, "CAHPS Survey for Accountable Care Organizations (ACOs) Participating in Medicare Initiatives: 2014 Medicare Provider Satisfaction Survey (English)," accessed May 18, 2014, http://acocahps.cms.gov/Files/SurveyInstruments/2014%20 CAHPS%20for%20ACOs%20Mail%20Survey%20(English).pdf.

23. David H. Maister, "The Psychology of Waiting Lines," in *The Service Encounter: Managing Employee/Customer Interaction in Service Businesses,* ed. John A. Czepiel, Michael R. Solomon, and Carol F. Suprenant (Lexington: Lexington Books, 1985), 113–124.

24. Centers for Medicare & Medicaid Services, "HCAHPS: Patients' Perspectives of Care Survey," accessed December 24, 2013, http://www.cms.gov/Medicare/Quality-Initiatives-Patient-Assessment-Instruments/HospitalQualityInits/HospitalHCAHPS.html.

25. Centers for Medicare & Medicaid Services, "Hospital Compare," accessed December 24, 2013, http://www.medicare.gov/hospitalcompare/search.html.

26. Centers for Medicare & Medicaid Services, "HCAHPS Survey," accessed December 24, 2013, http://www.hcahpsonline.org/files/HCAHPS%20V8.0%20Appendix%20A%20-%20 HCAHPS%20Mail%20Survey%20Materials%20(English)%20March%202013.pdf.

27. Centers for Medicare & Medicaid Services, "The HCAHPS Survey—Frequently Asked Questions," accessed December 24, 2013, http://www.cms.gov/Medicare/Quality-Initiatives-Patient-Assessment-Instruments/HospitalQualityInits/Downloads/HospitalHCAHPSFactSheet201007. pdf.

28. Quint Studer, Brian C. Robinson, and Karen Cook, *The HCAHPS Handbook: Hardwire Your Hospital for Pay-for-Performance Success* (Gulf Breeze, FL: Fire Starter Publishing, 2010).

# About Dr. Dorrah

Dr. Trina E. Dorrah is a board-certified internal medicine physician who practices as a hospitalist for Baylor Scott & White Health in Round Rock, Texas. She received her doctorate of medicine from Vanderbilt University School of Medicine. She then completed her internal medicine residency at the University of Alabama, Birmingham. Following residency, she received her masters of public health from the University of Alabama, Birmingham, and completed a fellowship in quality improvement through the Veteran Affairs National Quality Scholars program.

During her time in Birmingham, Dr. Dorrah realized her interest in quality improvement and patient satisfaction. After completing her training, Dr. Dorrah joined Scott & White Healthcare (now known as Baylor Scott & White Health) in Round Rock, Texas, where she was named medical director of quality. Through her time at Baylor Scott & White Health, she has led various improvement initiatives, but her passion lies in improving patient satisfaction. Dr. Dorrah works with providers to teach them how to improve their patient satisfaction scores. Teaching providers improvement skills to restore their excitement about patient satisfaction is something she loves to do. She truly believes satisfied patients lead to more satisfied providers. Dr. Dorrah hopes that, by sharing her insights and expertise, providers will embrace patient satisfaction and rediscover the joy of practicing medicine.